A FAMILIES' GUIDE TO

Health
& Healing

HOME REMEDIES FROM THE HEART

ALSO BY ANNA MARIA CLEMENT, Ph.D., N.M.D.

Relationships – Voyages Through Life

Children – The Ultimate Creation

A FAMILIES' GUIDE TO

Health & Healing

HOME REMEDIES FROM THE HEART
by Anna Maria Clement, Ph.D., N.M.D.

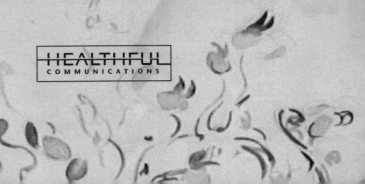

HEALTHFUL
COMMUNICATIONS

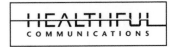

Healthful Communications, Inc.
Juno Beach Professional Building
13700 U.S. Highway One, Suite # 202A
Juno Beach, FL 33408
(561) 626-3293
www.healthfulCommunications.com

Contributing Editors
Brian R. Clement, Ph.D., N.M.D. and Lynn Komlenic
Healthful Communications

Publisher
Brian M. Connolly
Healthful Communications

Associate Publisher
Eric L. Zayes
Healthful Communications

Formulated by
George Kovac

Cover Art and Illustrations
Cecile Hubene

Typography
Yanileysi Bailes
Healthful Communications

ISBN 0-9771309-0-8

coolingtheplanet.com

♻ This publication is printed on recyclable paper with soy based inks and all the trees required to print this publication are replenished through **www.coolingtheplanet.com**.

"Life is an enormous opportunity to enjoy yourself and others more each day."

Brian Clement, Ph.D., N.M.D.

CONTENTS

CONTENTS

PLEASE NOTE

Before using this or any other health program consult with your physician. Everyone who utilizes this book — whether for self or another or others — must consider and implement the following provisos:

A. The individual — not any entity outside the individual, whether a family-member, friend, practitioner, pundit, group, book or system — is the source and continuity of all health, healing and self-maintenance. Therefore, this book — like all other external sources of information — is merely adjunct to each individual's absolute autonomy over her/his life and health.

B. Every person is unique. Therefore, before the application of any mode of procedure, all of the following facts about an individual must be considered and utilized:
    1. Gender
    2. Age
    3. Genetic history
    4. Health: Physical, mental, emotional & spiritual
    5. Physical condition
    6. Level of activity
    7. Diet
    8. Extraordinary circumstances (i.e., pregnancy)
    9. Climate, season and geographical location
    10. Schedule
    11. Occupation
    12. Individual conditions, circumstances and considerations

C. No mode of procedure can be useful — no matter how beneficial — unless it is utilized as properly directed.

ACKNOWLEDGEMENTS

First, I want to thank my parents, Eric and Margareta Gahns, who guided me into healthy living, and my husband, Brian, and our children, Daly, Danielle, Gail, and Blake for being my mentors.

I want to thank all of the people with whom I have worked — both my colleagues and our guests — at The Brandal Clinic and at The Hippocrates Health Institute. Their unwavering commitment continues to inspire me.

I want to give special thanks to the two exceptional women — Alma Nissen, the founder of the Brandal Clinic, and Ann Wigmore, the founder of The Hippocrates Health Institute — who gave me the confidence to live and to teach this natural healthy way of life.

I want to give special thanks to my husband, Brian, Co-Director of the Hippocrates Health Institute, and our friend George Kovacs, Communications Consultant to The Institute for their invaluable efforts in the compilation, writing and editing of this work, as well as the team at Healthful Communications for their invaluable editorial, design and marketing contributions.

And, my special thanks to Cecile Hubene for gracing our work with her splendid artistic contributions.

My love and best wishes to all of you who take this book to your hearth — your heart — and your home; may it help you and those in your life create magnificent vitality and well being.

FOREWORD BY VIKTORAS KULVINSKAS

Most of us are confronted by constant change imposed upon us by the external forces of our modern world— politics, technology, time, employment, retirement, and relationships to name just a few. These stresses tend to take us further away from nature and ourselves, and more into states of disease, suffering, distress and pain.

By contrast, this invaluable volume of self-assistance provided by Anna Maria Clement brings us back to nature and, in so doing, allows us to regain control of our lives and restore health. This comprehensive guide is a work that must not be kept on the shelf! Instead, it must be used in your daily life and with everyone whom you know. Not only is it a roadmap to wellness, it is a user's manual for the soul!

I had the good fortune of working for seven years with the estimable visionary, Ann Wigmore. We co-created **The Hippocrates Health Institute**, which pioneered the natural self-healing program that Anna Maria and her husband, Brian, have so masterfully nurtured and grown throughout the 20th century and now into the twenty-first.

For decades, our system of natural diet, positive attitude, and healthy exercise has benefited many thousands of people worldwide. I have been blessed to be involved with our development and prominence, a significant part of which has been Anna Maria's dedicated application of profound wisdom and international experience as a valued health professional. As you will see in this fine work, her contributions are not limited to **The Institute**; you can use them rewardingly and easily at home.

Health & Healing: A Families' Guide to Home Remedies From the Heart, is the ideal link between history and future, between nature and science, between institute and home, and between you and your health. So, it is appropriate that it comes from the accomplished Anna Maria Clement, who combines professionalism with caring, work with family, practicality with spirit, and optimism with sense. Her charm, good humor, and pleasant nature shine through in her writing and her presence. Now, they will illuminate your home, your health, and your heart.

This is a very practical book. It not only benefits your health and the health of your family and friends, but it also provides the means to do so easily and economically. The result of applying these time-tested principles is a healing organic lifestyle that promotes nutrition, health and longevity.

The Hippocrates Health Institute has contributed to our well being for decades; yet, this is just the beginning. With this glorious effort — and others in **The Hippocrates Series** — Anna Maria and Brian provide the means for all of us to live fulfilled, complete lives in harmony with nature and with our own best, most natural selves.

I am honored to write the foreword to this very important contribution to human welfare, lovingly offered by one of our finest contributors.

Viktoras Kulviniskas

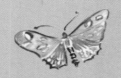

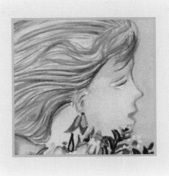

INTRODUCTION

Whole Health At Home

Historically, healing occurred in the home. Traditionally, healing was of little need because health was the hallmark of the home. Creating health in the home today, however, is increasingly difficult because of cultural changes and the fast pace at which we live, due in part to our technological age.

The world has become a global village; we rely upon strangers to grow our food, supervise our health, and heal our wounds. This is a new development. Our ancestors did these things for themselves, either individually, as families or in communities. But now we are faced with the challenge of restoring health...to our homes and ourselves. So, how can we make the best of both worlds? We can grow our own food, or support local organic farmers, and maintain our health by tending to physical, psychological and spiritual needs, all with the support of the most advanced information and technologies available today! This is the way to bring life back into our lives and our homes.

The Hippocrates Health Institute has led the development of life and dietary improvement in a clinical setting for more than half a century. As Health Administrator (and co-Director) of The Hippocrates Health Institute and previously as Director of **The Brandal Clinic** in Sweden, I have been privileged to implement and personally witness the many great benefits of using natural health remedies. It is now my great honor to share with you the foundation and essence of mental, physical, emotional and spiritual health, as well as a time-tested diet for everyone that is easy to understand and use in everyday life.

The founder of **Hippocrates**, Ann Wigmore, said about The Institute's mission: "We will help people to help themselves regain total health, naturally." We have remained true to this inspiration by educating people to be independent and responsible self-healers.

When we consider the many stresses that assault our hope and health, it is no wonder that illness on all levels — physical, mental, emotional and spiritual — has become commonplace. While our problems are both personal and global in nature, many of the solutions are home based. Yes, most of these problems can either be controlled, or neutralized, and even completely eliminated at home.

Many thousands of people throughout the world have attended The Hippocrates Health Institute to defeat disease, and thousands more have done so to delay aging, control their weight, improve their health, and elevate their lives.

It is critical to understand that a total reform in living is required in order to achieve complete health. This reform must start with you: your body, your mind, your emotions, thoughts and surroundings. And it must begin, remain and be maintained in the home.

We rarely consider our health during our daily activities; however, our priority should always be our health and the health of our family, both inside and outside the home.

Expecting others to maintain and, if necessary, improve our health is unrealistic and impractical. Instead, we must have and use the internal strength, increased awareness, and respect for our own resources to shape a full and balanced life.

I had the honor of being the Director of The Brandal Clinic, a respected treatment center for such autoimmune disorders as asthma, arthritis and Multiple Sclerosis. The Danish healer, Alma Nissen, who had been crippled by arthritis since her youth, founded The Brandal Clinic. Necessity forced her to learn to adapt a vegetarian diet that included plenty of garlic as medicine. She restored her own health fully. This was the first of my two experiences with the work of powerful women who, first, healed themselves and, then, created leading health institutes; the second was Ann Wigmore, creator of Hippocrates. When the physicians at Massachusetts General Hospital told Ann Wigmore that colon cancer would end her life, she chose not to accept that supposed finality. Instead, she instinctually began applying the basic principles that cause the mind, body, emotions and spirit to rejuvenate naturally.

The Swedish government so completely supported The Brandal Clinic that it not only referred all autoimmune related patients but it also funded research regarding various autoimmune problems. The results of this research indicated that more than 90% of the patients either improved significantly or healed completely.

As Health Administrator and co-Director of Hippocrates Health Institute, I have the opportunity to combine the best of two highly respected and proven traditions of natural healing; I am also able to use modern research and advanced methods of science and human potential, that are a result of an incredible global network, to help people achieve their greatest levels of health. As a mother, I have the practical opportunity of applying my experience and learning at home. Now, I offer you these years of experience and learning and the abundant knowledge of our predecessors as a pathway for recreating health in your home. May your journey to health be full of joy and light.

Anna Maria Clement, Ph.D., N.M.D.

(For more-detailed discussion of various subjects considered in this book, please see ***LifeForce*** and by Brian Clement, Ph.D., N.M.D., ***Living Food for Optimum Health***, and the other fine books in **The Hippocrates Series**.)

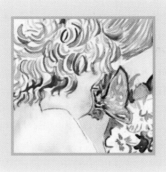

ONE

A Brief History Of
Traditional Medicine

Traditional medicine is just that — traditions or customs that are supported by many generations of use in homes, families and communities throughout the world. Today, people mistakenly use the word 'traditional medicine' when referring to 20th century modern medicine, when in fact, these newer practices have not been in use for very long nor stood the test of time. Traditional medicine involves not only solutions but also healthy living that eliminates the need for healing. The elements of traditional medicine are simple and complete; they include not only the physical products of nature (grasses, herbs, poultices, and fresh organic foods, to name a few,) but also the best elements of human nature — family and faith, as well as love, community, and commitment.

Our modern world is a global village, providing us with the great fortune of sharing healing traditions from every part of our world. We can learn from and use the wisdom and practices of the many ancient communities of Africa, Europe, the Pacific Ocean Nations and the Americas, as well as those of Asia, from the giant lands of India and China, to the small yet mighty of Tibet.

At the beginning of our history, we — explorers, creators, and nurturers — instinctively used all of the senses as a means of self-healing. Our senses enabled us to learn which environments were safe and healthy and which were not, as well as what foods were healthy to eat. The senses of sight, touch and smell led to regular self-cleansing, and the application of natural medications through the skin and massage, including aromatherapy. So, we used our senses to nurture and protect ourselves and — realizing their importance — we ourselves protected and nurtured them. So, it is from our natural core — the five senses – that we developed self-maintenance and self-healing, the essence of traditional medicine.

The most respected categories of traditional medicine include nutrition, proper exercise, positive mental activity, contemplation, rest and meditation, bodywork, aromatherapy, herbal medicine, naturopathy and homeopathy. And, in the spirit of these practices, they are often used in combination with each other. A very important part of whole health and natural healing is accepting all valid approaches from all legitimate sources. This is supported by the inclusive wisdom of Paracelsus' writing in 1520: "I went not only to local doctors, but also to nurses, bath keepers, other learned physicians, women, and everyone who practices the art of healing; I went to chemists, to monasteries, to nobles, to common folk, to the experts, and to the simple." It is beautiful and sound advice and today, with the use of modern technology, we can gather and assemble this collective wisdom to our greatest benefit.

More and more people are finding modern medicine ineffective and are returning to traditional methods. There are even enlightened medical professionals who are using traditional medicine whenever possible.

Modern medicine has its challenges: the methods tend to be complicated and often take us out of our home, both physically and virtually. And, just as the body is the home of our being, so is our home the center of our activities. We are most comfortable there, so let us use it to serve all of our needs — physical, mental, emotional, and spiritual. Look inside before you go outside for solutions, acceptance and validation and you will find that health has always been simple: live positively, eat well, be harmonious, and share wholeheartedly.

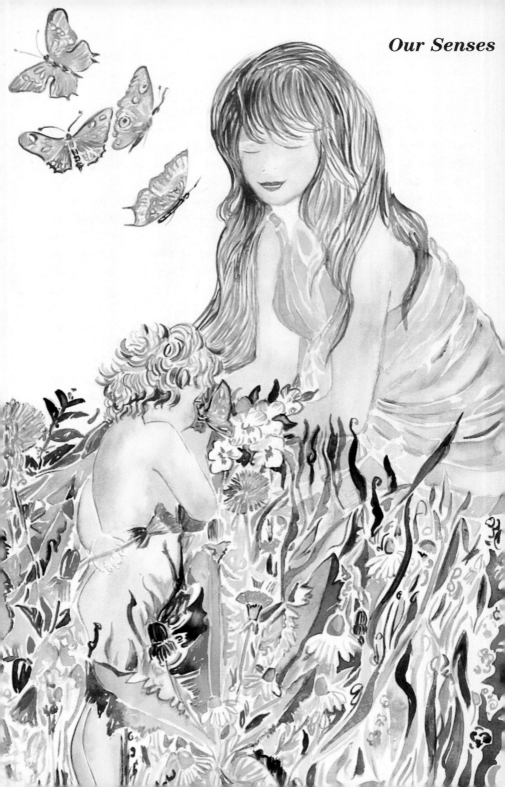

Natural living and self-healing are as old as humanity, having been advocated by Hippocrates (the father of Western medicine) and his fellow healers in all cultures. Even those who preceded him, including such founders of universal medicine as Maimonides, Shen Nung and Sushruta spoke of the power of natural methods. Throughout history, there have been many insightful natural healers. These noble practitioners established traditions of natural health in every part of the world, in every society, and in every community.

Ancient traditional methods, which are now being recognized in western cultures, are widely documented and used extensively in other cultures today. Native American healers, for example, not only extracted the medicine of Echinacea (commonly used now to support immune function) from plants but also respected and cultivated the soil in which it grew. Ancient South American herbalists gave us ayahuasca (a natural chemical curative not commonly known today, but used in a wide variety of disorders. Other traditions such as rebirthing (established in New Zealand) and healing wands, made of stones, leaves and oils (originating in Australia,) have been employed successfully for a variety of diseases over the years. And for many centuries now, the world has been familiar with the various and significant contributions of Asian medicine such as acupuncture and herbal medicine.

Traditional African medicine deserves special attention, not only because it has been such an important part of worldwide health maintenance, but also because of its spiritual connection to whole health. In fact, traditional African healing is based upon the broader concept that a malady is much more than physical; it is an indication that ones life is out of balance and in violation of nature and life itself. This greater perspective compels the healer to look at the various internal and external relationships of the patient, both personal and environmental, to find the cause and the solution of the condition. The ultimate purpose of an advanced healer is to reconnect the patient with the spiritual essence of life — the essence that Asians traditionally call "chi". There is this logical, natural, and absolute connection between these two highly respected ancient traditions of healing.

During the 18th and 19th centuries, various communities and movements of natural living and diet were established throughout the world. However, over the years and for a variety of reasons we have mostly abandoned nature and moved away from a natural way of living. In spite of technological advances, we are still faced with unprecedented disease, some of epidemic proportions, like cancer and obesity. The only logical way to move forward is to go back . . .back to nature.

Our journey back to natural living is easy if we grasp the loving hand of Mother Nature and appreciate her bounty. This book is the map for that journey and the evidence of her appreciation.

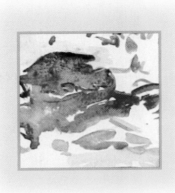

TWO

Hydration:
You Need Pure Liquids

W e can live without food for many weeks; we can live without water for only three days! Like oxygen, water is necessary for life. It is necessary both inside and outside the body, and equally important to our skin as it is to our cells and our blood. So, drinking pure water is not enough (and, these days, not even easy). We must bathe and apply water on and to ourselves in all possible ways, while taking time to purify and protect our valuable resources.

Approximately 70% of our body is water, as is approximately 70% of the Earth's surface; this is another example of the harmony of natural design. After oxygen, water is the most important basic element of life. Our best sources of pure water are steam-distilled water and molecularly organized filtration. Pure water is essential to healthy cells, the foundation of life; it is the best conductor of the electric current of the body, serving as an unrestricted highway on which all cells can move and interact freely. This

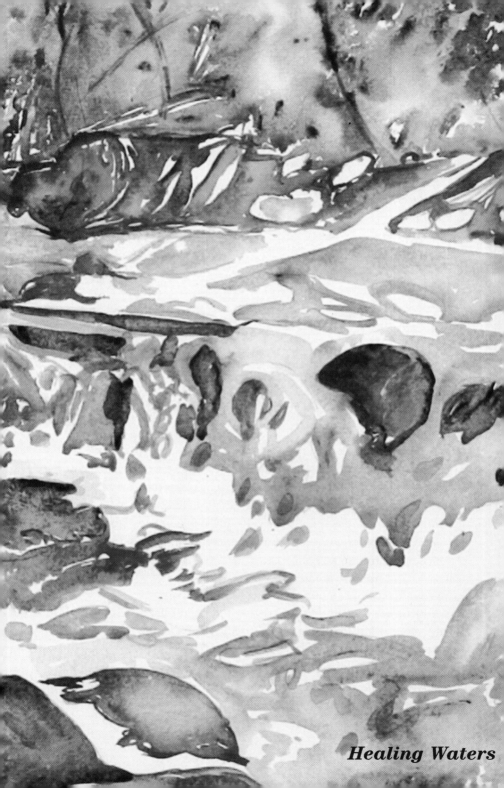

Healing Waters

open flow charges the meridian system (electrical roadway), thereby increasing our cell's ability to create a powerful self-protective electric shield, which prevents radical electrons (free radicals) from destroying healthy cells. Free-radical damage is the cause of disease, premature aging, and most other internal damage to the body.

Major symptoms of water deficiency are dry skin and mouth, memory loss, delusion, and possible death. Drinking too much water, on the other hand, may cause edema, congestive heart failure, and respiratory failure. Similarly, drinking water that contains toxic chemicals and other impurities, not only prevents the positive interaction of the electrical, hormonal, and metabolic systems of the body but it also promotes mutagenic (cancer-causing) activity.

Soaking in pure water that has been enriched by organic minerals, oils and herbs has always been an excellent method of healing and relaxation. Natural waters have been used frequented by both the healthy and the fragile. The body, mind, emotions and spirit alike are calmed and refreshed by these therapeutic waters. Minerals are essential to the healing effects of all-natural spring baths such as sulphur springs, which are famous for helping osteoporosis and arthritic disorders. Other minerals in these waters — depending on their composition, quality and quantity — provide additional medicinal and soothing effects. Natural-water resorts exist throughout the world; find them and enjoy them!

Because of its chemical likeness to human blood, bathing in ocean water provides great benefits. Bathing in water containing 5-8 cups of dissolved pure sea salt in a standard bathtub assists circulation, nerve function, healthy skin, detoxification, and relaxation.

Water used in our living, work and educational environments can be both pleasant and relaxing. Fountains, waterfalls and technically generated sounds of natural water calm the neurological system and promote the release of endorphins, creating positive brain chemistry and stimulating the development of leukocytes in the immune system.

Before pollution, all rainwater was naturally distilled. For a long time, the only water that people used was collected rainwater. Our ancestors knew that our waterways had biological pollutants; so, they avoided water from those places whenever possible. Today, we drink and cook and bathe with water from many polluted sources.

The pollution of our water by poisonous chemicals limits our choice of healthy water to molecular organization and distillation. These two forms of water purification eliminate poisons and pollutants (including MTBEs, the most toxic substances generated by mankind thus far.) No other forms of filtration or cleansing destroy these health and life-threatening compounds completely.

Hydration of the cells of the body is crucial to the bio-chemical and electrical functioning of every system. If you drink too little pure liquid, the systems of your body decline, beginning with a loss of electrolytes, the possible result of which is death! Coffee, sugar-filled carbonated drinks, alcohol, and salt-filled beverages are not only dangerous to our health but they also drain the body of the fluid that is essential to it.

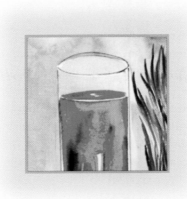

THREE

Raw Living Herbs
And Grasses In Healing

T he **Hippocrates Health Institute** is named after Hippocrates, a great ancient Greek healer. It is appropriate that this book about **The Institute's Home-Health Program** focus on the natural healing elements — such as living herbs and grasses— which Hippocrates and his counterparts in every culture on every continent used in the tradition of maintaining health.

From our beginnings, long before Hippocrates and other popular healers, we were in harmony with nature, enjoying her healing gifts and applying them to ourselves, our children and even our pets.

The medicinal use of herbs is many thousands of years old and includes all of humanity, Chinese and Asian people, Egyptians and other Africans, Greeks, Romans, and natives of the Americas and the lands of the Pacific Ocean. A Greek physician named Discorides wrote the first detailed list of herbs, covering more than 400 healing plants. His work, presented in four books, was published during the time of Nero and used for more than two centuries throughout Europe.

Living herbs and grasses have always been paramount to health and healing. They have also been used in many other traditions, such as in perfumes and cosmetics, as garnishes and flavoring for foods, pest control, and traditions of spirituality. We have created countless balms, tonics and cures by combining various living herbs and grasses into unique blends that provide relief. It is important to take note of *The Doctrine of Signatures*, an ancient belief that plants resembling specific parts of the body could be used to heal those same parts, when affected by disease. For example, lungwort— also called pulmonaria— was named in both instances for its resemblance to diseased lungs because of its white-spotted leaves.

When possible, it is best to grow or gather everything that you put into and onto your body. But, at a certain point in our development, that became impossible. First, families farmed together; then, people formed communal groups to share the bounty of nature. Now, in our modern global village, we have the good fortune and ability to rely on our fellow humans for our natural food and medicine. Even though they may live far from us, they are a part of our extended but very real family.

It is easy and pleasant to grow most herbs and grasses; but we must be aware that they require individual care and cultivation. Proper combination and application of herbs is critical; they must be appropriate for each condition and individual. This requires knowledge of the length of growth, season of collection, duration of effectiveness, and the unique properties and limitations of herbs individually and in various combinations. Lastly, all herbs must only be used — whether at home or institutionally — in small amounts and for minor ailments when you do not have access to expert medical advice.

THE ALPHABET OF HERBS

Medicinal herbs are the main medicine of 4/5 of the world's population. Western cultures remain the 1/5 of the population that prefers "modern" pharmaceuticals; however, approximately 1/4 of all pharmaceutical medicine consists exclusively of herbs. With the exception of nuclear medicine, all pharmaceuticals have plant-based origins.

Schools of herbology have developed at various times and in various locations. Most respected among them is the Asian tradition, which spans several thousand years. The practitioners of this well documented science have demonstrated that every ailment has a natural remedy. But, people in 'the West,' still consider herbal medicine as an alternative treatment rather than primary medicine. In addition, many people make a distinction between pharmaceutical medicine and the herbal type, believing that they can use herbs without concern, care or restriction. Herbs are medicine and must be given the same consideration and used with the same discipline as pharmaceuticals, which are sadly, often misused. Furthermore, combining herbal medicines, herbal medicines with pharmaceuticals, and various pharmaceuticals with each other is potentially very dangerous. Overuse, misuse and abuse of pharmaceuticals is a serious problem. Pharmaceutical medicine can be helpful when properly used, but only after all herbal medicinal options— the most natural means of healing— have been considered with the advice of a knowledgeable practitioner. It is rare that you would need to consume any herb for long periods of time. Of course, there are exceptions, for example, natural hormones for women, ginkgo biloba for cranial and ventricular problems, and cranberry extracts for kidney infections and bladder problems.

Some seasonings and herbs, like mints, oregano and camomile, are not dangerous, even if they are used as condiments throughout a lifetime. Exceptions are various salts and black peppers as well as herbs and seasonings that are most frequently used as medicine.

We, at Hippocrates Health Institute have established a healthy pattern of use for medicinal herbs. Take medicinal herbs for three days, and then suspend use for the next two days. In addition, do not take them every eighth week– or every 50th-56th day. This provides better results than repeated ordinary use.

Common herbs like echinacea are best when you are exposed to infection at home, work, or school. Once you have been infected, echinacea is of no value; an herb such as osha or, temporarily, silver nitrate (colloidal silver) is better. Aloe Vera can be used daily, because it is in the rare category of medicinal food–herbs, which means it is both food and medicine. Within the family of medicinal food-herbs, there are

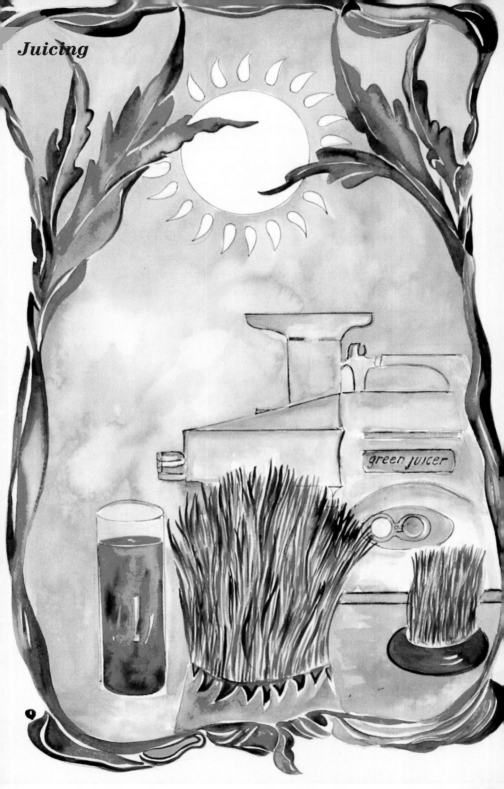

exceptions. Cayenne, for example, should not be used in large amounts over a long period of time.

The origins of herbal medicine can be traced to the African continent. Unfortunately, both that history and the history of Native American herbology are almost completely lost because of the tragic destruction of these populations and the brutal disregard for their traditions and artifacts. Health and healing have specific individual histories based upon geography and culture. As such, the residents of each region and of each individual group developed their own medicinal systems to combat disease.

The variety and availability of herbs internationally is awesome. For example, throughout Europe, healing plants found in the north— for example, Lapland— are different from those of the same variety harvested in the south. Similarly, there are hundreds of varieties of medicinal herbs in Australia that are unique not only to that continent but to each region as well. In South America and in the islands of the South Pacific, herbs are plentiful and used regularly for nutrition, health and healing.

Seasons and altitudes are as important an influence for herbs as they are for certain plants. For example, while nettles are everywhere on earth, they develop mostly during the spring season of a particular region. Their blood purifying properties are welcome after a long, dark winter. Certain plants, such as dandelion-flower, can be found only at higher altitudes during the hottest days of summer; so, residents at those cooler altitudes can harvest them for their blood building benefits. Accordingly, many herbs can be found only at lower altitudes, such as desert aloe.

Consuming fresh raw herbs is best; however, seasonal limitations often leave us with the sole choice of utilizing dry varieties. When using dried herbs for medicinal purposes internally, it is best to make sun tea from them first. Use a container of pure water and add herbs as appropriate. Place the container on the windowsill for 24 hours; make sure that your window remains closed. If you want warm herbal teas, be sure that you do not heat this liquid at a temperature above 42 degrees Celsius or approximately 115 degrees Fahrenheit. There are exceptions to the raw or sun tea methods of herbal use. Use dried or non-gelatin-encapsulated powders and herbal pills (that have not been heated), or cook a combination of herbs to create a salve or tincture, which results in a new natural chemistry. In addition to the herbs' primary properties, the new tincture has its own medicinal properties that provide great benefits. Adding small amounts of fresh herbs to your juices enhances the already powerful effects of these beneficial and nutritious liquids. For example, the juiced combination of gingerroot and green vegetable aides in the digestion of their nutrients, regulates the thermostat of the body, and calms the stomach and intestines.

If you must rely on processed herbs, do your best to find those that are in liquid glycerine. These extracts are much more likely to be digestible than other forms. They are also preserved by the glycerine, which protects their medicinal fluids from oxidization (loss of potency).

Following is an alphabetical list of herbs that are most often used to enhance health and healing. Whenever possible, use them in their fresh and raw state and evaluate and use your choices with the guidance of a health professional.

HERBS	MEDICINAL ATTRIBUTES
Acacia	Fatigue (Epstein-Barr Virus)
Agrimony	Laryngitis; sore throat
Angelica	Respiratory/bronchial; anti-viral
Ashwaganda (*Indian Ginseng*)	Enhances the immune system; increases energy; reduces stress
Basil	Mildly sedative; antiseptic; relieves nausea
Bearberry	Skin problems (cystitis, eczema, psoriasis)
Betony	Exhaustion; stress
Black Cohosh	Circulatory problems; hormone adjuster
Boneset	Influenza; aches
Borage	Depression; general health
Buchu	Skin problems (cystitis, eczema, psoriasis)
Burdock-root	Acne; boils; blood cleansing
Butcher's Broom	Alzheimer's Disease; senility; heart-disease; gangrene; circulatory problems
Catmint	Colds; catarrh; colic; bronchitis; flatulence; sinusitis
Caraway	Colic; intestinal inflammation
Cayenne	Colds; improves blood circulation; chilblain

HERBS	MEDICINAL ATTRIBUTES
Celery-seed	Arthritis; gout; fever(s)
Chamomile	Asthma; digestion; indigestion; headache; insomnia; stress; gall bladder problems; bites; fluid-retention; menstrual problems; abscesses
Chaste Tree	Pre-menstrual symptoms; menopausal problems
Chickweed	Eczema; bites/stings
Cinnamon	Colds; fever
Circu Formula	Circulatory problems
Cleavers	Pre-menstrual symptoms; blood cleansing; Kidney cleansing
Coltsfoot	Cough; whooping cough
Cone-flower	Tonsillitis; skin irritations; mouth ulcers; acne; athlete's foot; thrush; immune function
Comfrey	Eczema; bruises; cuts; sprains
Couch Grass	Pre-menstrual symptoms; urinary cleansing
Cramp Bark (European Cranberry Bush)	Relaxant; sciatica; cramps; menstrual problems
Damiana	Impotence
Dandelion	Liver maintenance; diuretic; biolaxative;
Dandelion-leaf	Constipation; gall bladder problem; rheumatism
Dandelion-root	Boils; fluid retention; juice combats warts; improves functioning of the liver and bowels
Devil's Claw	Gout; circulatory problems
Dill	Colic; flatulence
Dong Quai	Endometriosis
Elder	Cysts; coughs; catarrh; rheumatism; sciatica
Elderflower	Acne; sinusitis; stings; circulatory problems
Eucalyptus	Allergies; catarrh; emphysema; pneumonia respiratory problems
Evening Primrose	Eczema; women's hormonal imbalance
Eyebright	Asthma; Eye disorders; Hay fever

HERBS	MEDICINAL ATTRIBUTES
Fennel	Colic; flatulence; fluid retention
Feverfew	Headache; migraine; arthritis; natural insect repellant; reduces temperature
Geranium	Cardiovascular benefit; liver enhancer
Gentian	Depression
Ginseng *(FOR MEN ONLY!)*	Impotence; enhanced sexual potency energy enhancement
Hops	Relieves stress; promotes sleep
Horse Chestnut	Hemorrhoids; varicose veins
Horse-radish	Benefits lungs and circulation; blood cleanser
Horsetail	Prostate problems; urinary incontinence
Hyssop	Colds; coughs; insomnia; nasal congestion
Iris-flower	Cartilage; joints; ligaments; membranes; tendons
Juniper	Digestion; kidney function; blood cleanser
Kava Kava	Stress; depression; anxiety
Kohlrabi	Anti-mutagenic; ulcers; digestion problems
Lady's Mantle	(Pre-)Menstrual problems; Menopausal problems
Lavender *(Lavender oil)*	Antiseptic; fainting (equilibrium sustainer); rheumatism; acne; asthma; diarrhea; sciatica; spasms; whooping cough; boils; bites/stings; cold-sores
Lemon Balm	Anxiety; insomnia; nervous system disturbance acidity; heartburn; indigestion; flatulence; menstrual problems; bites/stings
Lime-blossom	Stress; digestion; pain; heart functioning; circulatory problems; varicose veins
Linseed *(flaxseed)*	Constipation; digestive disorders
Marigold	Bites/stings; wounds; burns; conjunctivitis; athlete's foot; eczema; hemorrhoids; thrush
Marshmallow-leaf	Bronchitis; coughs
Meadowsweet	Acidity; arthritis; diarrhea; fibrositis; heartburn; stomach problems; fluid retention; rheumatism

HERBS	MEDICINAL ATTRIBUTES
Myrrh	Sore throat; tonsillitis; athlete's foot
Nettle	Arthritis; internal bleeding; blood disorders; Skin conditions; circulatory problems; eczema; psoriasis; gout
Oatstraw	Depression; sciatica; nervous system stability; impotence
Orris	Throat infection; bladder problems
Parsley	Anemia; arthritis
Passion-flower	Stress; sedative; sleep
Pau d'arco	Bed sores; boils; cancer; canker; Immune disorders
Penny-royal	Flatulence; nausea; headaches
Peppermint	Catarrh; digestion; headache; sinus-problems; fainting; nausea; vomiting
Pilewort	Hemorrhoids
Plantain	Bites/stings
Quinoa	Builds red blood cells; strengthens the neurological system
Raspberry-leaf	Brain function; gall bladder problems Laryngitis; sore throat
Red Clover	Blood cleanser; bites/stings; eczema; psoriasis
Ribwort	Diarrhea
Rosemary	Depression; digestion; headache; nervous system
Rue	Epilepsy; eczema; psoriasis; ointment form for eyes and throat
Sage	Laryngitis; mouth ulcers; tonsillitis; menopausal problems
Saw Palmetto	Prostate problems
Slippery Elm	Acidity; heartburn; stomach problems; boils
Sorrel	Diuretic; renal (kidney) tonic
St. John's Wort	Anti-inflammatory; nervous system restorative; psychological disorders
Tarragon	Toothache; anti-mutagenic

HERBS	MEDICINAL ATTRIBUTES
Tea Tree	Burns; antiseptic; anti-microbial
Thyme	Bronchitis; coughs; diarrhea; laryngitis; mouth ulcers; tonsillitis
Uva Ursa	Kidney congestion; bladder congestion; backache; prostate; gonorrhea; syphilis
Valerian	Sedative; tranquilizer; insomnia; nerves; menstrual problems
Vervain	Depression; neuralgia; convalescence
Wall-flower	Arterial elasticity; cardiovascular function
White Deadnettle	Menstrual problems; prostate problems
White Horehound	Bronchitis; coughs
Willow Bark	Fibrositis; gout; pain
Wild Indigo	Cold sores; herpes
Witch Hazel	Hemorrhoids; cold sores; cuts; nosebleed; varicose veins
Xanthium	Hepatitis; colds; influenza (flu); SARS; other microbial infections
Yarrow	Colds; diarrhea; dysentery; as an astringent;
Yarrow-root	Circulatory problems; cuts; nosebleed; Chicken pox; fluid retention
Yellow Dock	Bites/stings; blood cleansing; psoriasis
Zingiber	Fights microbes and mutagens; vomiting; nausea
Zingiber Offcinale	Controls raised temperature; chilblain; fever; alleviates bronchitis; morning sickness
Ginger; Gingerroot Jamaican Ginger	Rheumatism; prevents motion sickness

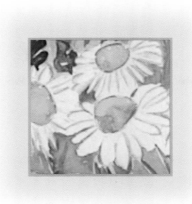

FOUR

Nutritional And Topical Use Of Living Herbs And Edible Weeds

A s we know from our years of work at the Institute, raw living food is the cornerstone of healthy living. As Hippocrates said, "Let thy food be thy medicine and thy medicine be thy food." It is logical that these direct and immediate products of nature, that provide us with abundant nutrition internally, can also be applied successfully to our bodies externally. To quote Ann Wigmore, "you should be able to eat whatever you put onto your skin."

Among the most versatile healing tools used throughout the world is wheatgrass, the application of which is developed and emphasized daily at **The Hippocrates Health Institute**. This superfood has become one of the most popular natural health foods today; and it has always been among the most effective. Its nutritional excellence and versatility derives from its similarity to the hemoglobin of our blood. When consumed orally

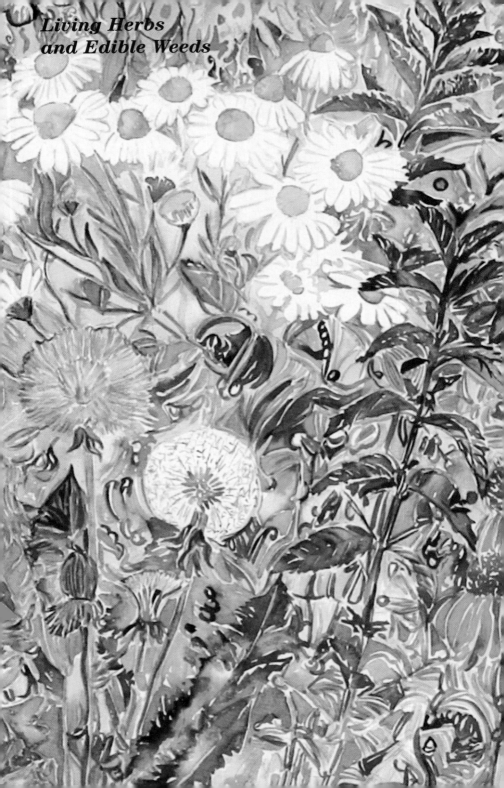

Living Herbs
and Edible Weeds

or implanted anally, this blood-building dynamo helps to rid the body of debris, while strengthening its cells and organs. This miraculous substance not only purifies and heals the vaginal and rectal canals, it helps to prevent premature graying and unnatural hair loss. Externally, it can be applied therapeutically to the eyes and used as a natural bandage on the skin. Daily use of wheatgrass juice is one of the best ways to increase your family's health.

Following is a brief list of natural solutions (including wheatgrass or course) to various health-problems:

PROBLEM	SOLUTION	USES
Arthritis of Extremities	*Wheatgrass-in-packing*	Soak a cotton sock with 6 ounces (180 milliliters) of wheatgrass juice; place on affected area; cover with plastic bag and a dry sock.
Asthma	*Eucalyptus-leaf*	With mortar and pestle, press the fresh leaves into small open pieces; add 2 oz. (60 milliliters) of flax-oil; let it sit for 24 hours. Consume 5 drops of the preparation 4 times per day. Repeat process until you achieve relief.
	Garlic (Please see the chapter entitled, "Garlic: Nature's Powerhouse".)	
Burns *(Including Sunburn)*	*Aloe-vera leaf*	Break a leaf; apply the gel from the open leaf to the burn.
	Ice	Apply ice to burn.
	Baths; showers	Take cold baths and/or showers.
Cough(s)	*Raw Aloe and Grapefruit-seeds*	Break open 30-50 grapefruit seeds; let sit in 4 ounces (120 milliliters) of raw aloe vera for 12 hours in the refrigerator. Consume 1-3 tablespoons (5-15 milliliters) as needed.
Diarrhea	*Raw mint leaves and green clay*	Take 4 ounces (120 milliliters) of edible clay powder; add 2 ounces (59.14 milliliters) of pure water and one ounce (30 milliliters) of finely cut fresh mint leaves. Let sit for 3 hours; consume 1/2 ounce (15 milliliters) as needed.

PROBLEM	SOLUTION	USES
Earache	*Garlic-oil*	Prepare one part pressed garlic and two parts room-temperature cold-pressed uncooked olive oil. Saturate cotton ball and place it into the ear canal.
Eyewash	*Wheatgrass-juice*	Massage around the eyes lightly. In an eyecup, mix 1/2 ounce (15 milliliters) of strained wheat-grass juice and 1/2 ounce of pure water. Look upward. Put eyecup to eye for 15-30 seconds. (Might burn slightly.)
Fever	*Dry ginger-powder*	Only once or twice per week when you are healthy. When you are feverish, you can use it once per day: Dissolve one cup in hot bath water. Soak for 15-20 minutes. Rinse with a cold shower. Promotes perspiration.
General Detoxification	*Wheatgrass juice*	Drink 2-4 ounces (60-120 milli-liters). Implant 4-6 ounces (120-180 milliliters) rectally, after enema.
	Sea-salt *Epsom salt* *Kosher salt* *Crystal salt* *Celtic sea-salt*	Once or twice per week: Dissolve one cup in hot bath water. Soak in water for 15-20 minutes. Rinse with a cold shower. (Add one pound of baking soda to neutralize radiation, chemicals and heavy metals.)
	Dry ginger-powder	Only once or twice per week when you are healthy; when you are impaired, use it once or twice per day: Dissolve one cup in hot bath water. Soak for 15-20 minutes. Rinse with a cold shower. Promotes perspiration.
	Dry-skin brush	Immediately before showering: Using circular motions and straight strokes toward the solar plexus, rub your entire skin surface vigorously. (Stimulates the lymphatic and circulatory systems.)

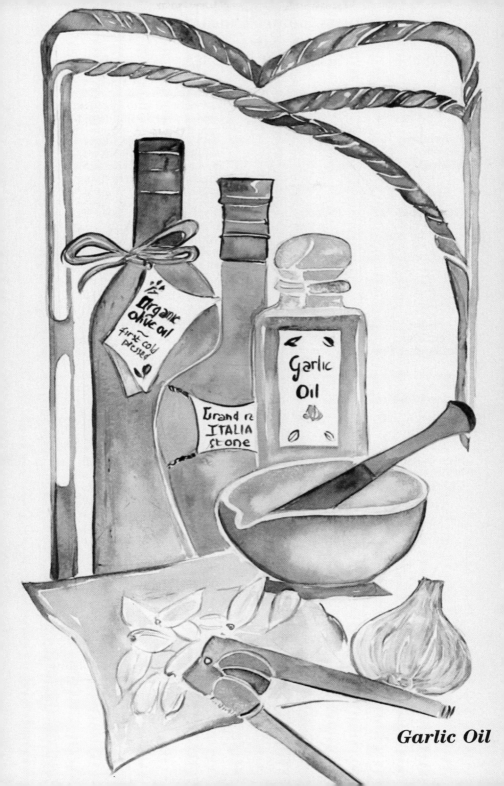

Garlic Oil

PROBLEM	SOLUTION	USES
Hair/Scalp: Dandruff;	*Wheatgrass juice*	Massage six ounces into scalp. Cover head with shower cap; leave on for 15 minutes; rinse.
Psoriasis; Dry/Oily Scalp	*Neem*	Juice or press neem leaves; apply the extract directly to affected areas. (You can buy natural neem extract and apply similarly.)
Headaches	*Enema and implant*	Drink at least 2 quarts (2.5 liters) of pure water daily. Cleanse the colon: Take a one-quart (1.25 liters) pure-water enema; follow with wheatgrass implant.
	Magnesium	Drink 1 tablespoon of liquid magnesium in 8 ounces (240 milliliters) of pure water or any raw juice.
Infections; Colds and Flu	*Osha and Silver Nitrate*	Drink six drops of each herbal Tincture in pure water several times per day.
Liver-Detoxification	*Castor oil*	Rub onto skin directly over liver. Then, place a cloth made of natural fiber onto liver; place hot-water bottle onto cloth, and leave for 30 minutes.
Measles; Mumps: Chicken pox	*Silver nitrate, raw aloe and camphor*	Place 6 ounces (180 milliliters) of raw aloe into bowl; add 25 drops of silver nitrate and 1 ounce (30 milliliters) of camphor (preferably raw). Stir for 3 minutes. Apply thoroughly on infected area(s). For mumps, rub directly into the skin covering the throat. And drink 1 ounce (30 milliliters) of this mixture twice per day while the condition persists.
Nosebleed(s)	*Fenugreek sprout juice*	Juice 8 ounces (240 milliliters) of fenugreek sprouts; recline; apply the extract directly into affected nostril(s) with a dropper. Apply pure cotton to the nostrils to maintain and contain the healing liquid.

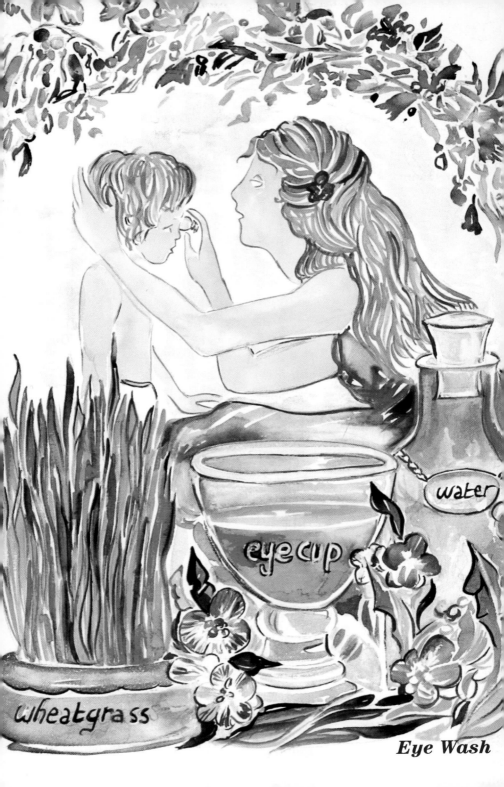

wheatgrass

eyecup

water

Eye Wash

PROBLEM	SOLUTION	USES
Osteoporosis	*Tiger-balm and silica or horsetail-tea*	Place 2 ounces (60 milliliters) of tiger-balm into bowl; add 20 drops of silica or 1/2 ounces (15 milliliters) of horsetail herbal tea; combine; apply to affected areas.
Pneumonia	*Fresh grass juice and horseradish-extract* **CONSULT PHYSICIAN!**	For every 3 ounces (90 milliliters) of barley-grass juice, mix 1/4 ounce (7.5 milliliters) of horse radish-juice. Consume Consume 4-6 times per day.
Rejuvenation	*Cold shower Stimulating essential oils*	Finish every shower or bath with a shower of cold water. Dip one finger into your chosen essential oil and place some under each nostril and one drop on the middle of your forehead and on the palm sides of your wrists several times per day.
Relaxation	*Dry ginger-powder*	Once or twice/week: Dissolve one cup in hot bath-water. Soak for 15-20 minutes. Rinse with a cold shower. Then, pat yourself with a towel, but leave yourself slightly moist; wrap yourself into towels; place yourself under the covers of your bed; relax, and sleep, if possible. This process promotes perspiration and soothes neurological function and the brain.
Skin: Eczema; Psoriasis	*Oregano and hemp oil*	Topical application of poultices as appropriate. Mix 4 ounces (120 milliliters) of fresh Oregano juice or finely chopped oregano with 4 ounces of hemp oil; leave for 4 hours; apply moderately to affected areas.
	Wheatgrass poultice	Make poultice using 2 ounces (60 milliliters) of wheatgrass juice and enough pulp to absorb the juice atop the gauze. Apply poultice to the affected area;

continued on next page

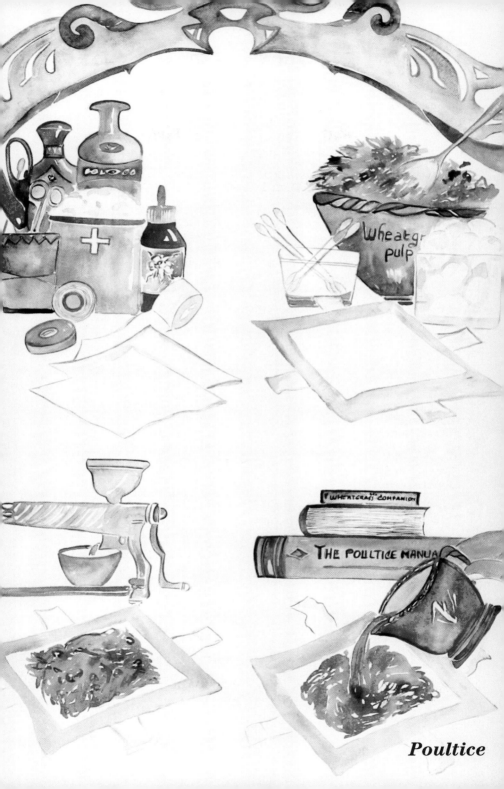

Poultice

PROBLEM	SOLUTION	USES
continued from previous page	*Wheatgrass poultice*	cover it with a bandage; secure it with tape. Leave it on affected area for approximately 8 hours.
	Garlic (Please see the chapter entitled, "Garlic: Nature's Powerhouse".)	
Tumors	*Wheatgrass poultice* SEE "WHEATGRASS POULTICE" UNDER "SKIN"	
Tumors; Open sores	*Garlic oil*	Apply a mixture of one part pressed garlic and two parts Olive oil to compress and apply it to any open wound as a disinfectant. Wrap with gauze. (The oil can remain usable in the refrigerator for four days.)
Urinary Problems	*Raw apple-cider vinegar and Cranberry seed powder*	Mix 2 ounces (60 milliliters) of raw apple-cider vinegar with 4 tablespoons (20 milliliters) of cranberry seed powder. Drink every 5 hours during the day — **DO NOT INTERRUPT REGULAR SLEEP.**
Vaginal Discharge; Fibroid tumors; Cysts; Yeast-infection(s); Herpes; Post-Menstruation	*Wheatgrass juice douche*	Put 2 ounces (60 milliliters) of wheatgrass juice into 2 ounces of pure water. Add enzymes and probiotics as needed. Implant with bulb-syringe.
Warts; Skin Tags	*Cedar oil/juiced cedar leaves*	Dip q-tip into selected fluid; apply directly to affected area. **USE EXTREME CAUTION IN AND NEAR EYES!**

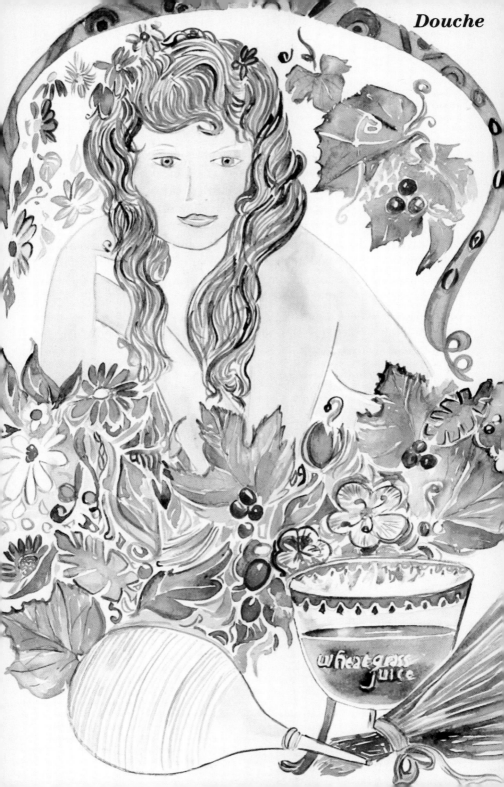

CAYENNE

Traditionally, cayenne has been used to coagulate the blood that results from wounds. Use as follows: apply ground cayenne powder directly to the affected area and cover with a bandage. It will sting slightly. Cayenne calms ulcers, lowers blood pressure, improves circulation, and helps to clean and maintain the cardiovascular system. **Capsicum**, the medicinal extract of cayenne pepper has even more power to combat all of these maladies. Using this hot pepper and its extract, you can reduce the intensity of the symptoms of the common cold and *influ*enza. Many other kinds of peppers (such as black and white pepper) contain irritating oils that aggravate the gastrointestinal and digestive system; so, they should not be used. Cayenne—this miraculous herb and food— was first used in Africa, the birthplace of civilization.

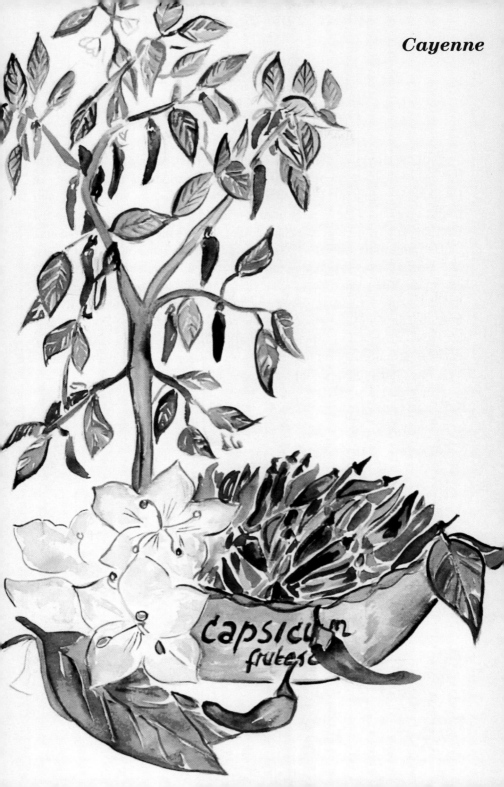

Cayenne

capsicum
frutescens

ALOE VERA

Both the energy of the sun and the medicine of nature are contained in this tropical sun-drenched plant. You will experience a great variety of benefits by adding this hot weather member of the cactus family to your health program. Aloe Vera is used worldwide to heal burns, cleanse the body, improve digestion and elimination, activate the immune system and, most importantly, strengthen the body in its war against disease. It is best and most effective when taken in its raw, fresh form, either internally or externally. The second best means of application is frozen aloe, while the third is whole-leaf bottled in its raw state. Aloe Vera has been used as an intestinal implant in cases of diverticulosis, Crohn's Disease, colitis, leaky-bowel syndrome, and other similar afflictions. For health maintenance, consume 2 ounces (60 milliliters) of raw or frozen aloe vera per day and/or 4 ounces (120 milliliters) of bottled aloe vera.

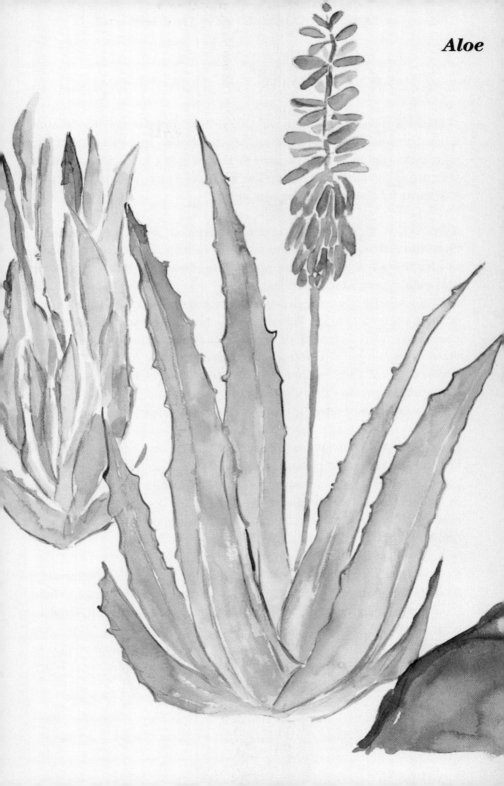

Aloe

PURCHASING LIVING FOOD AND OTHER ITEMS FOR THE HEALTHY HOME

Markets throughout the world stock fresh organic and biodynamic foods daily; these nutritional powerhouses are filled with essential natural substances. Equipment to prepare these raw living foods is available in both actual and virtual retail stores as well as at **The Hippocrates Health Institute**, by phone, e-mail or regular mail.

Sprouts— First, we have the organic biodynamic seeds, nuts, grains and beans that can be grown into extraordinary food sources. You have thousands of choices, all of which have unique aspects of the full range of the nutrients required for superb health.

Vitamins, minerals, trace elements and proteins are just the basic elements of these nutritional foods. All advanced scientific research indicates that chlorophyll, pure water, fiber, oxygen, enzymes, hormones and phyto-chemicals are other vital elements contained in these foods. As research and knowledge progress, we will discover other elements that are as important as the ones that we know.

Sprouts are the most nutritious foods grown on land.

Sea-vegetables— are the most-nutritious food(s) in our oceans –and include nori, dulse, arame, hijiki, wakame, and other edible algae. These foods contain plentiful minerals and trace minerals as well as amino acids that contribute to the building and functioning of every cell of the body. Most diets do not contain sufficient quantities of minerals to sustain good health. So, we must eat sea vegetables regularly to have and maintain full health.

Fresh-water algae— *green and blue-green types* are the most nutritious foods in fresh waters (rivers, lakes, streams, brooks, and springs.) These foods not only have the most protein but they are more than 50% amino acids, by weight. They are also the plants that contain the most chlorophyll as well as rare trace elements and rare DNA-building ingredients. In addition, the polysaccharides and chlorophyll-related pigments in fresh-water algaes stimulate stem-cell development.

Sprouts, sea-vegetables and fresh-water algae are at the heart of **The Living-Food Diet**; they are the most-nourishing food on earth.

Vegetables— of all types are an essential part of the Living Food banquet; they add variety and nutrition and stimulate our senses with their colors, textures and tastes. The ideal way to enjoy these foods is when they are fresh from the garden. Most of us purchase bio-organic food after it has been stored and shipped, and when it has lost much of its nutrition and electrical charge. Most of the nutritional frequency of these foods is lost just hours after harvesting. Although these vegetables are not as dynamic as a growing sprout or freshly harvested vegetables, they are still much better for you than most other choices.

Fruit— We have the good fortune to enjoy hundreds of kinds of fruit. The significant water content of these mineral-rich foods is a wonderful complement to the body, which, itself, is approximately 70% water. When you are healthy, no more than 15% — by weight — of your diet can be ripe organic fruit. When you are unhealthy, however, have no fruit at all, because fruit contains too much fructose, a type of sugar that feeds and worsens all disease.

Juice— All healthy juice is made of two basic sources — organic and bio-available plants and fruits. Plants from which juices are made include: grasses, sprouts, leafy vegetables, herbs, flowers, and, on occasion, leafy and wild greenery. We eat and drink these superb products of nature— either whole or juiced— not only for their obvious bodybuilding values but also because of their medicinal value. Fruit-based juices contain smaller amounts of nutrients and vitamins but higher levels of enzymes and minerals than those that we get from most green plants. It is important to always add pure water to pressed ripe bioorganic fruit juices to dilute the sugar (fructose) in them. Remember, too much fructose can compromise your health.

Juices made from grass, sprouts, and green vegetables are a significant part of the Hippocrates diet. These chlorophyll-rich green juices contain basic building blocks of vitamins, amino acids, minerals and various phytonutrients. Drinking them regularly helps your blood cells thrive. There is only one chemical difference between chlorophyll and the hemoglobin in human blood: the center molecule in blood is iron; while in chlorophyll it is magnesium. Research has proven that drinking juices made from organic/ bio-available sprouts and green vegetables every day improves and maintains your health and healing.

THERAPEUTIC JUICES

Juicing is the best way to get the most nutrition from plants; it eliminates the fiber from plants so that their nutritional components are easily absorbed. Juice is essentially the nutritional version of the blood that builds and strengthens our bodies. Sunlight nourishes all physical forms of life, and plants store sunlight. As a result, juices are among the most important supplemental foods because of their combination of nutritional vitality and captured sunlight. Condensed nutrition derived from plants provides nourishment from multi-vitamins, minerals, trace minerals, oxygen, enzymes, hormones, and phytonutrients. Drinking juices 15 minutes or less after they have been extracted is very important if we want to take advantage of all of their nutritional advantages.

The juices of grasses, sprouts, flowers and fresh herbs can be added to the juices of vegetables and fruits. The Institute's research indicates the possibility that drinking undiluted fruit juices might feed disease. We, at Hippocrates encourage the use of green vegetable and sprout juices and discourage the use of diluted fruit-juice. A healthy person should drink a combination of approximately 10% fruit juice and 90% pure water. Those who have health problems should not have any form of fruit juice or the sweet juice of vegetables such as carrots, and beets; they contain too much sugar. Similarly, you should add very little juice from herbs and/or flowers, because of their strong medicinal effects. When you juice vegetables, fruits, herbs and flowers, be sure to strain the juice so that all of it can be mixed without considering food combining. Some combinations of juices increase healing effects, creating better results. Even the healthiest person gains great benefit from the drinking fresh green juices daily. Two 12 or 16-ounce (360-480 milliliters) sprout-vegetable-juices twice per day are an important part of **The Hippocrates' Living-Food Program.**

Additionally, drink two ounces (60 milliliters) of wheat, spelt, kamut and/or barley juice — or any combination of them — twice per day. Drinking green juice and grass juice daily gives your blood and its cells the basic nutrients and purification that they need.

We have been drinking juices from the beginning of history. Energy, strength, cleansing, healing, hydration, as well as the building and maintenance of the electrolyte system and the two fluid-based systems of the body— the kidney system and the respiratory system— are the main benefits of drinking these enzyme-rich liquids. Following is a list of our favorite therapeutic juices:

THERAPEUTIC VEGETABLE JUICES, FRUIT JUICES AND SPROUT JUICES
(USE ONLY ORGANIC/BIO-AVAILABLE FOODS)

ALFALFA-SPROUT JUICE: Creates **fibrin,** the structural foundation of the human cell. Strengthens **blood**; this, in turn, builds strong **tissue,** reduces **edema,** and strengthens **muscle** and **bone**.

ANISE SPROUT JUICE: Good for the **respiratory** and **cardiovascular** systems. Also enhances the development of the **t-cells** of the **immune system**.

ASPARAGUS JUICE: Assists **renal (kidney) function,** neutralizes **kidney stones** and **bladder stones**, and regulates **urinary flow**.

ARTICHOKE JUICE: Enhances the functioning of **renal, immune** and **digestive** systems.

BEET JUICE: Consumed in small quantities is a **blood purifier** and **blood strengthener, varicose vein reducer**, and **arterial** and **cardiovascular** cleanser.

BROCCOLI SPROUT JUICE: Its **phytonutrient** content enables it to reduce the potential for **mutagenic growths,** including **cancer**. Facilitates **healthy and consistent elimination**.

BRUSSELS SPROUTS: Contain **proteins** that help to generate **insulin,** improving **pancreatic function** and combating **digestive disorders**.

THERAPEUTIC VEGETABLE JUICES, FRUIT JUICES AND SPROUT JUICES
(USE ONLY ORGANIC/BIO-AVAILABLE FOODS)

CRESS (CREST) SPROUT JUICE: Builds **blood** by multiplying **red blood cells**; decreases **toxins** in the **respiratory system**; acts as an **anti-fibroid, anti-cystic, and anti-carcinogenic agent.**

CUCUMBER JUICE: Benefits **respiratory, joint, ligament,** and **kidney** functioning; increases **dermal (tissue-) elasticity.**

CAULIFLOWER JUICE: Improves the functioning of **skeletal, digestive** and **eliminatory** systems.

CELERY JUICE: Facilitates **dermal detoxification and circulation.** Reduces **uric acid**; improves **electrolyte function**; detoxifies the system of the effects of **nicotine** and **caffeine**; promotes **dermal (skin-) flexibility.**

CABBAGE SPROUTS: Help to combat **irritated and inflamed digestive tract, ulcers,** and **osteoarthritis/osteoporosis.**

CAYENNE-PEPPER-SEED SPROUTS: Resists **heart attack, stroke** and faulty **circulation,** and benefits those who have had conditions of **the cardiovascular and circulatory systems.**

CANTALOUPE GREEN SPROUTS: Increases sperm and egg production; combats **excess blood sugar,** whether low or high.

DIKON RADISH JUICE: Blood thinner— maintains **electro-magnetic functioning of the solar plexus.**

DANDELION JUICE: Creates **red blood cells**; strengthens **gums and teeth**; assists **healthy skeletal and dental bone development.**

ENDIVE JUICE: Improves **vision**; reduces the potential for and the severity of **cataracts**; creates strong **ventricular tissue.**

FENNEL-SPROUT JUICE: Builds **white and red blood cells**; increases **digestive enzymes.**

FENUGREEK-SPROUT JUICE: Combats **body odor**; fights **gastrointestinal disorders**; regulates **blood sugar** in both **hypoglycemia** and **diabetes.**

THERAPEUTIC VEGETABLE JUICES, FRUIT JUICES AND SPROUT JUICES
(USE ONLY ORGANIC/BIO-AVAILABLE FOODS)

GARLIC-SPROUT JUICE: Fights **cancer, ulcers, parasites, amoebae**; improves **protein levels in the blood.**

HORSERADISH JUICE: Consumed in small amounts, removes **excess mucous; diuretic;** helps to counteract **colds and flu.**

IRIS-FLOWER JUICE: Builds **ligaments, tendons, cartilage;** strengthens **joints;** improves **membrane development.**

JERUSALEM ARTICHOKE: Regulates **blood sugar** problems; builds **energy.**

KALE-SPROUT JUICE: Its **calcium** and **sulfur** are perfect **bone builders** and **digestive aides.**

LILY-FLOWER JUICE: Builds **capillaries;** strengthens **vision** and **hearing;** assists the **h-cell** development of the **immune system.**

LILY-FLOWER JUICE: Builds **capillaries;** strengthens **vision** and **hearing;** assists the **h-cell** development of the **immune system.**

LEEK-JUICE: Combats **cancer, mutagens, ulcers, parasites.**

LETTUCE-JUICE: Subtle **aphrodisiac, mood enhancer, skin restorer, hair restorer.**

MANGO-SEED-SPROUT JUICE: These **enzyme rich plants** promote **healthy digestion and elimination,** while building a reserve of **vitamins and minerals** to create **healthy and stable organs.**

MUSTARD-SEED-SPROUT JUICE: Dissolves **hemorrhoids;** eliminates **mucus** from the **respiratory system;** reduces length and impact of **colds and in***fl***uenza.**

NASTURTIUM JUICE: Builds the **immune system, fighter cells** and **eosinophils;** purifies the **lymphatic system** and the **bloodstream.**

ORANGE-SEED-SPROUT JUICE: Powerful **phytonutrients** to combat **viral and bacterial disease;** assists the **neuronal functions** of the **brain.**

THERAPEUTIC VEGETABLE JUICES, FRUIT JUICES AND SPROUT JUICES
(USE ONLY ORGANIC/BIO-AVAILABLE FOODS)

ONION-SPROUT JUICE: Anti-mutagenic; purifies **liver, gall bladder, spleen, small intestine** and **large intestine**; builder of **immune cells** and **red blood cells**.

PAPAYA-JUICE (Including seeds): Rarely found **fibrin** content enhances **gastric, digestive and pancreatic juices** to **build blood platelets and reduce external and internal scar tissue**.

PARSLEY-JUICE: Minimizes the pain of **menstrual cramps**; fights **coronary disease, cataracts, conjunctivitis, glaucoma**; improves **vision, cardiovascular functioning**, and **blood count**.

PEPPER-SEED-SPROUT-JUICE, (RIPE RED, YELLOW, PURPLE): Reduces **bloating, flatulence, colitis**, and **colic**. Rich in **vitamin C**; strengthens **metabolism**, specifically of **the heart**; reduces the potential of **microbial infection**.

POTATO (WHITE) JUICE: (After extraction, leave for 2 minutes so that unwanted starch is separated from consumable juice.) Increased **minerals,** especially **potassium,** assist **cardiovascular function** and **kidney function.** Specifically effective against **arthritic and osteoporotic conditions.**

QUINOA-SPROUT JUICE: (These sprouts should be harvested and juiced on the fifth day of sprouting.) The combination of **prominent protein content** and **minimal glycemic properties** of **quinoa sprouts** makes them a **super fuel** that **energizes all bodily functions**, thereby **increasing stamina, strength and muscle development**.

RADISH-SPROUT JUICE: Increases **digestive capability**; reduces **fibroid and fibroid cystic growths**; acts as a **powerful agent against mutagens and cancer.**

RAW SAUERKRAUT JUICE: Improved **dermal (skin-) elasticity and appearance**; cleanses and builds **digestive organs**; enhances the **probiotics** in **the gastrointestinal tract** which, in turn, **strengthens immune cells**.

RED-PEPPER-SEED-SPROUT JUICE: These **vitamin-C-rich** powerhouses are the most **effective** means to neutralize, and even prevent, **viral infections**. They also help to prevent **blood clots** and **strokes**.

THERAPEUTIC VEGETABLE JUICES, FRUIT JUICES AND SPROUT JUICES
(USE ONLY ORGANIC/BIO-AVAILABLE FOODS)

SORREL-JUICE: Enhances **healthy skeletal and dermal development**; creates **greater bone density** in the lower extremities.

SPINACH-JUICE: Prevents **anemia, convulsions, neural disorders, adrenal dysfunction**; also builds **red blood cells** to cleanse the **liver**, thereby improving **immune function**.

STRINGBEAN-JUICE (Green, purple): Regulates **blood sugar** (both **diabetes** and **hypoglycemia**) via **insulin-stimulation**; develops **proteinase (protein digesting enzymes)**.

SWEET-POTATO SPROUTED JUICE: These juiced greens build **healthy tissue**, fulfill various **nutritional deficiencies**, and create **elasticity of ligaments**.

TOMATO-SEED-SPROUT JUICE: Increases the **metabolism**, reducing excess **weight**; reduces fluid in **edema**; the **lypine content** in its **phytonutrients** attacks **cancers** of the **prostate**, **breast** and **colon**; combats **hepatitis A, B, C.**

TOMATO-JUICE (Unsprouted): Contains minimal amounts of **lypine**; although it is effective in the **reduction of cancers of the colon, prostate, and breast** and in combating **hepatitis A, B, C**, it is less effective in doing so than tomato-seed-sprout juice. **It also detoxifies the liver and gall bladder.**

TURNIP-GREEN JUICE: Builds **bones; facilitates digestion**; reduces potential **colon polyps** and **hemorrhoids**.

UVA URSA (BEARBERRY) SPROUT JUICE: Eliminates excess **mucus**; resists **microbial infection**; a **diuretic, astringent, mucilage-antiseptic, disinfectant**.

VIOLET-FLOWER JUICE: Consumed in small quantities, this **spleen stimulating** fluid assists the production of **healthy red blood cells, fingernails and toenails**.

THERAPEUTIC VEGETABLE JUICES, FRUIT JUICES AND SPROUT JUICES
(USE ONLY ORGANIC/BIO-AVAILABLE FOODS)

WATERCRESS-JUICE: Increases **hemoglobin** to prevent **anemia** and **chronic low blood-pressure**; strengthens **joints, cartilage, tendons, ligaments**; helps to reduce **tumors** by **improving circulation**.

XANTHIUM-SEED-SPROUT JUICE: This anti-viral juice fights **hepatitis A, B, C, HIV, colds, flu, SARS**, and other **microbial infections**.

YAM-SPROUT JUICE: These succulent greens function as **hormonal balancers** and suppliers of everything from **progesterone** to **testosterone** to **DHEA**; this juice minimizes **the effects of PMS, menopause, mood swings,** and increases **sex drive**.

YELLOW-SQUASH JUICE: This liquid is filled with **bone building minerals**; it also acts as a **diuretic** and **relieves constipation**.

YUCCA-ROOT-SPROUT JUICE: The juice of these green leaves elevates endurance and **energy** levels and stimulates the **immune function** of **glucocytes** to **combat all forms of disease**.

ZINGIBER-OFFCINALE- (Ginger; Jamaican ginger) SPROUT-JUICE: Harvested as a small sprouted plant and then juiced, it helps to regulate the **internal thermometer** — including **slightly raised temperature** — to **combat microbes and mutagens**. It also assists in the prevention of **motion sickness**.

OTHER BUILDING FOODS

NUTS— almonds, filberts, pine-nuts, macadamias, walnuts, pecans, pistachios (but not peanuts and cashews,) all in raw and sprouted form, are very important to your health, because they are easily made into loaves, croquettes, burgers, sauces, and other nutritious and familiar "food" forms.

SEEDS— sunflower, pumpkin, sesame, hemp, flax— are lighter than nuts, and they are used as often in the development of familiar preparations.

Nuts and seeds replace the more filling foods that have been removed from your former diet. Because nuts and seeds are heavier than most other natural foods, they should be eaten in moderate amounts and regulated based on a person's metabolism. Those who have sluggish metabolism and slow digestion should eat just small amounts of nuts and seeds; those with faster metabolisms and digestion and, typically, a more active life (including pregnant women and nursing mothers) can eat slightly more.

AVOCADO— this unique food, that is both fruit and vegetable, is also heavier than the average natural food. Like nuts and seeds, someone transitioning to The Living-Food Diet often consumes too many avocados. While this response is natural, it is mostly due to an emotional need rather than a nutritional one, and will pass quickly.

Dehydrated foods are essential to starting and continuing The Living-Food Program. By drying vegetables, nuts, seeds and prepared dishes, you can create the taste and feeling of cooked food. Enzymes and nutrients remain in dehydrated foods, as long as they are dried at 115 degrees Fahrenheit or less; this maintains their nutritional value beyond that of cooked foods. Including a great variety of delicious dehydrated foods will help you maintain a positive and happy relationship with the living foods program.

The healthy person can also consume small quantities of cooked organic/bio-available foods. If you are in the process of rebuilding your health, maintain a 100% raw/living-food diet. Otherwise, cooked food can be added, but no more than 25%, by weight, of what you eat. Most people who eat cooked food, but follow a raw living-food diet, choose to have less than that.

Research by **Hippocrates Health Institute** has proven that proper diet and healthy living protect the immune system from microbes and mutagens. Those who maintain a 75%+ raw-vegan diet are significantly protected from disease. When that percentage drops below 75%, however, the immune system weakens, allowing a greater chance for disease and illness. In our research, a 10-15% decrease in raw living food results in a 47% reduction of immune function.

Your ability to build and maintain your body depends to a great extent on the amount of nourishment that you provide to your cells. Those who choose foods from The Hippocrates Program possess and maintain increased health and vitality. "Foods" that are not part of The Program damage health, steal energy, cause disease, and shorten life. Be sensitive, not only about the foods you choose, but also about your relationship with it; avoid overeating, binge eating, and other bad habits and you will enjoy and appreciate food on the highest levels and as intended by nature.

BACH FLOWER-REMEDIES

Bach Flower Remedies are another category of homeopathic medicine. Dr. Edward Bach discovered that flowers have frequencies that cause emotional balance in people. His approach to healing is summarized by Frances Wheeler in the following passage from ***The Bach Flower Remedies***:

> Dr. Bach taught that the basis of disease was to be found in disharmony between the spiritual and mental aspects of a human being. This disharmony, to be found wherever conflicting moods produced unhappiness, mental torture, fear, or lassitude and resignation, lowered the body's vitality and allowed disease to be present. For this reason, the remedies that he prepared were for the treatment of the mood and temperament of the patient, not for his physical illness, so that each patient becoming more herself could increase her own vitality and so draw from an inward strength and an inward peace the means to restore health.

During the Twentieth and Twenty-first Centuries, Dr. Bach's remedies have been used more and more throughout the world. These remedies were available only in alcohol; today, they are also available in distilled water. Following is a list of some **Bach Flower Essences** and the problems that they address:

BACH FLOWER ESSENCES

EMOTION(S)	BACH FLOWER REMEDY
Anxiety; despair; fear(s); loneliness; hypersensitivity:	**Agrimony**
Delusion(s); depression; fear(s); insomnia; nightmares; stress; tension:	**Aspen**
Anger; antipathy; intolerance; irritability; stress; tension:	**Beech**
Anxiety; depression; fatigue; intimidation; melancholia:	**Centaury**
Anxiety; indecisiveness; uncertainty:	**Cerato**
Desperation; fear; insanity; instability; stress; tension:	**Cherry Plum**
Impatience; inattention:	**Chestnut Bud**
Anxiety; fear; fretfulness; possessiveness; self-pity:	**Chicory**
Apathy; despair; exhaustion; faintness; melancholia; numbness:	**Clematis**
Despondency; moroseness; obsessiveness; self-loathing:	**Crab Apple**
Despondency; failure; inadequacy:	**Elm**
Anxiety; depression; melancholia:	**Gentian**

BACH FLOWER ESSENCES

EMOTION(S)	BACH FLOWER REMEDY
Despair; indecisiveness; melancholia; resignation:	**Gorse**
Antipathy; anxiety; self-pity; worry:	**Heather**
Antipathy; despair; vexation; violence:	**Holly**
Despair; melancholia; pessimism:	**Honeysuckle**
Apathy; fatigue; insecurity:	**Hornbeam**
Impatience; insecurity; intolerance:	**Impatiens**
Fear; indecisiveness; insecurity; pessimism; procrastination:	**Larch**
Fear; insecurity; nervousness; tension:	**Mimulus**
Anxiety; despair; melancholia:	**Mustard**
Despondency; futility; instability:	**Oak**
Anxiety; exhaustion; fear; gloom:	**Olive**
Despondency; guilt; self-criticism:	**Pine**
Apprehension; anxiety; tension:	**Red Chestnut**
Anxiety; despair; fear; panic:	**Rock Rose**
Anxiety; self-criticism; stress:	**Rock Water**
Anger; indecisiveness; insecurity; instability; unpredictability:	**Scleranthus**
Despondency; grief; shock; tension:	**Star of Bethlehem**
Anguish; despondency; fear:	**Sweet Chestnut**

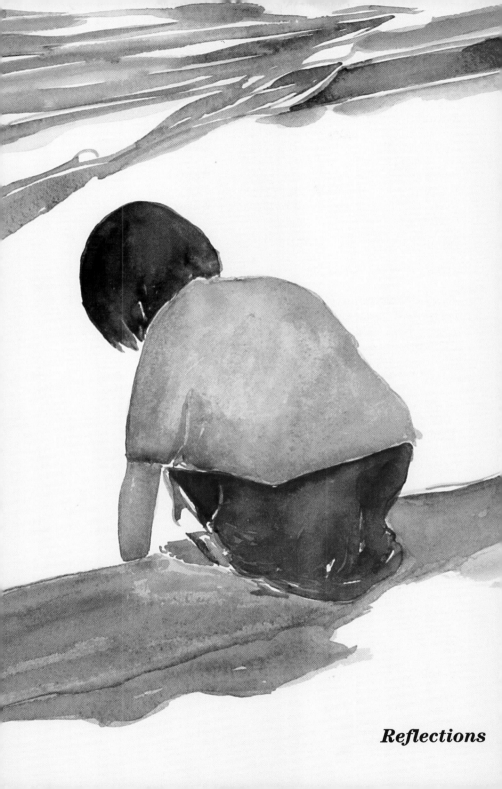

Reflections

BACH FLOWER ESSENCES

EMOTION(S)	BACH FLOWER REMEDY
Exhaustion; intolerance; tension:	**Vervain**
Authoritarianism;inflexibility:	**Vine**
Frustration; hypersensitivity:	**Walnut**
Indecisiveness; intolerance; sadness:	**Water Violet**
Anxiety; confusion; inattentiveness:	**White Chestnut**
Indefiniteness; insecurity:	**Wild Oat**
Apathy; exhaustion; gloom; resignation:	**Wild Rose**
Argumentativeness; bitterness; desperation; resentment:	**Willow**

FOR ALL EMOTIONAL EMERGENCIES AND STRESS: RESCUE REMEDY

In my own life, **Rescue Remedy** has been of great help during the natural birth of my children and instances of stress.

As you can see, the essences and extracts of living herbs and edible weeds are among nature's greatest gifts to us. We can apply them both internally and externally to heal us; use them to keep yourself healthy, so that you never need to be healed.

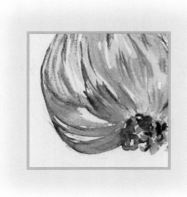

FIVE

Garlic: Nature's Powerhouse

G arlic is among nature's greatest gifts to us. It has been used world-wide throughout history as an anti-viral, anti-fungal, anti-bacterial, anti-parasitic, anti-amoebic, anti-cancerous, anti-spirochete medicinal, as well as for inflammations and catarrh. Civilizations revered its effectiveness so profoundly that they wore garlic traditionally to defend themselves from every form of evil. It is the most extensively used healing food among people of Latin descent, while the Romans and Egyptians cherished garlic so much that they regarded it as a delicacy.

Researchers at Harvard University conducted a study that revealed that garlic selectively isolates and completely destroys cancer cells. Garlic contains all of the essential amino acids, which are the building blocks of proteins.

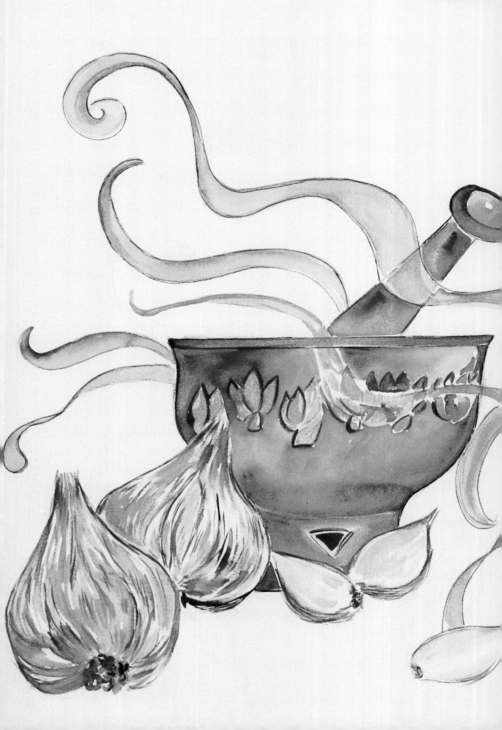

Dr. Christine Nolfi, founder of the Danish clinic called "Humlegarden" created the term, "living food". In addition to the raw vegetarian diet that she prescribed for her patients, the staple was the frequent daily use of garlic.

In my work both in Europe and North America, I have witnessed the potent cleansing powers of garlic. When all other possibilities fail to heal wounds and infections, garlic serves to do so. There is no doubt that applying pressed garlic soaked in cold-pressed oil to infected areas is the most effective way to clean, heal and disinfect. Likewise, garlic oil is an excellent balm for external wounds, ulcers, gangrene, and other eruptions. It is also helpful in assisting post-operative healing.

Garlic can have powerful and sometimes irritating effects on your tongue and stomach. Therefore, consume 1-2 cups of flax-water (20% flaxseed: 80% pure water; left for 24 hours before use) before you eat raw garlic. A Scandinavian recipe for the consumption of raw garlic is to combine pieces of garlic with pieces of an organic apple. The pectin of the apple coats the mouth, thereby rendering the liquid extract of the garlic palatable.

Garlic is a standard remedy for arthritis, asthma, gout, emphysema, heart problems, excess cholesterol, high blood pressure, infections, parasites, and many other disorders. It is truly a wonder food, in and for your palate and on and through your skin.

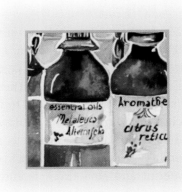

SIX

Essential Oils: Aromatherapy

A romatherapy is an important component in the tradition of herbal medicine. While aromatherapy is part of the history of many cultures, Middle-Eastern cultures in particular are given credit for its formal discovery and development. More than a thousand years ago, Arabic people invented a way of distilling oils to create substances that had both delightful aromas and healing properties...the word 'essential' hinting at the importance of these natural healing elements. Many cultures since then have contributed significantly to the development of aromatherapy. The French, for example, have long regarded the making of perfumes as an art form. Their great love for aroma has resulted in both hygienic and medicinal applications of fragrances worldwide.

Essential oils are very concentrated: as many as 5,000 roses are used to make just 5 milliliters— 1 tablespoon— of pure Oil of Rose! Be careful though, too much of a good thing, even an essential oil, might irritate your skin or have toxic effects. Because of the expense and quantity of natural resources used in making essential oils, they must be used cautiously and wisely.

Like many things with healing properties, oils can lose their effect with frequent use. To receive the greatest benefit from oils, rotate them after using any one oil or group of oils for ten days. Also, be aware that certain combinations of oils may cause sensitivities such as headaches or even nausea. When combining oils, mix two, three or, at most, four at a time. Used sensibly, essential oils are a wonderful addition to The Living-Food Program. When taking essential oils internally, use only 100%-pure organic oils under the guidance of a trained health care professional.

Following is a list of essential oils and their benefits. Traditionally, essential oils were regarded as combined elements of balance; so, they were discussed in terms of yin or yang. Yin is big and broad, soft and subtle, producing greater potential. Yang is concentrated power and outwardly moving energy producing positive limitations.

THE ABBREVIATED ALPHABET
OF AROMATHERAPY

BENEFIT(S)/RELIEF FOR...	ESSENTIAL OIL
Despair; discouragement:	**Angelica (YIN)**
Asthma; arthritis; bronchitis; colic; gout; laryngitis; sores:	**Benzoin (YANG)**
Abscesses; acne; bronchitis; cancer; cystitis; depression; diphtheria; fevers; infections:	**Bergamot (YANG)**
Cataracts; cholera; diarrhea; dysentery; heartburn; nausea; toothache; vertigo; vomiting:	**Black pepper (YANG)**

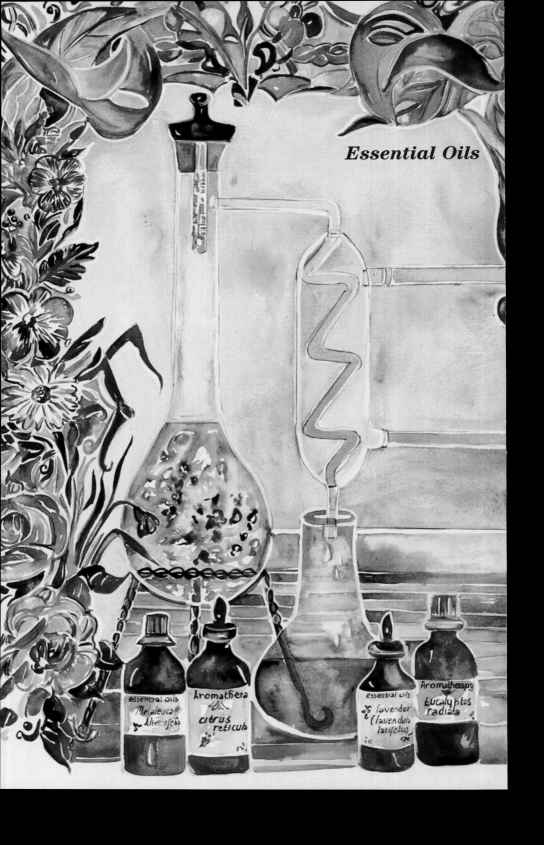

Essential Oils

THE ABBREVIATED ALPHABET
OF AROMATHERAPY

BENEFIT(S)/RELIEF FOR...	ESSENTIAL OIL
Allergies; anemia; colitis; convulsions; depression; earache; hysteria; insomnia; irritability; jaundice; menopausal problems; migraines; rheumatism; urinary stones; ulcers; vaginitis; wounds:	**Camomile (YIN)**
Acne; bruises; burns; cholera; constipation; depression; gout; heart-failure; inflammation; insomnia; tension; pneumonia; shock; sprains; tuberculosis:	**Camphor (YIN)**
Relaxant; brain-balancer; boils; convulsions; infections:	**Clary sage (YANG)**
Asthma; hemorrhages; hemorrhoids:	**Cypress (YIN)**
Calming agent; mild sedative:	**Dill (YIN)**
Purifier, invigorator; enhances concentration; catarrh; cystitis; diabetes; emphysema; gallstones; herpes; malaria; measles; neuralgia; pediculosis; scarlet fever; sinusitis; typhoid fever; wounds:	**Eucalyptus (YIN)**
Alcoholism; hiccoughs; kidney-stones; insufficient milk of nursing mothers; nausea; obesity; pulmonary infections:	**Fennel (YANG)**

THE ABBREVIATED ALPHABET
OF AROMATHERAPY

BENEFIT(S)/RELIEF FOR...	ESSENTIAL OIL
Comforting; self-integrating; catarrh; deep, peaceful calm; gonorrhea; laryngitis:	**Frankincense (YANG)**
Confidence; emotional strength:	**Ginger (YANG)**
Deep, calm breathing; hormonal balance; dermatitis; influenza; otitis; pertussis; scrofula; pertussis; urinary stones; wounds:	**Hyssop (YANG)**
Confidence; security; openness:	**Iris (YIN)**
Stress-minimizer; anxiety; depression; hoarseness; frigidity; impotence; tension:	**Jasmine (YANG)**
Arteriosclerosis; cirrhosis; diabetes; dropsy; rheumatism:	**Juniper (YANG)**
Anti-depressant; mental clarity:	**Kava Kava (YANG)**
Conjunctivitis; convulsions; cystitis; diphtheria; epilepsy; fainting; neurasthenia; paralysis; pertussis; sunstroke:	**Lavender (YANG)**
Confidence; elevation of spirit:	**Lemon (YANG)**
Arthritis; dysmenorrhea; tics:	**Marjoram (YANG)**
Allergies; colds; depression; dysentery; indigestion; migraine:	**Melissa (YANG)**

THE ABBREVIATED ALPHABET
OF AROMATHERAPY

BENEFIT(S)/RELIEF FOR...	ESSENTIAL OIL
Confidence; healing; strength; gingivitis; hemorrhoids; thrush; tuberculosis; ulcers; wounds:	**Myrrh (YANG)**
Elation; euphoria; fulfillment; joy: Depression; diarrhea; hysteria;	**Niaouli (YIN)** **Neroli (YANG)**
Insomnia; palpitations:	**(Orange-blossom)**
Enthusiasm; intensity; vigor:	**Oregano (YIN)**
Anxiety; depression; wounds:	**Patchouli (YANG)**
Mental fatigue; neuralgia; paralysis; ringworm; shock:	**Peppermint (YANG)**
Anxiety; fear; stress:	**Pettigrain (YIN)**
Autonomy; calmness; self-control:	**Quinine (YIN)**
Hepatic congestion; impotence; insomnia; sterility; vomiting:	**Rose (YIN)**
Anti-depressant; humanity; humility; arteriosclerosis; cirrhosis; colitis; epilepsy; pertussis:	**Rosemary (YANG)**
Relaxant; heightened sensuality cystitis; laryngitis; nausea:	**Sandalwood (YANG)**
Antibacterial; antifungal; antiseptic; antiviral; purifier; elevates potential:	**Tea-tree (YANG)**
Confidence; hopefulness; security:	**Uva Ursa (Bearberry) (YIN)**

THE ABBREVIATED ALPHABET
OF AROMATHERAPY

BENEFIT(S)/RELIEF FOR...	ESSENTIAL OIL
Anxiety; stress-relief; calm:	**Vanilla (YANG)**
Impenetrability; peacefulness; solitariness:	**White pine (YIN)**
Confidence; inner strength; resolve:	**Xanthium (YANG)**
Euphoria; invigoration; aphrodisiacal; depression; frigidity; impotence:	**Ylang Ylang (YIN)**
Concentration; consciousness:	**Zucchini-flower (YIN)**

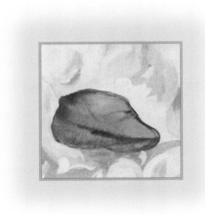

SEVEN

Serious Solutions
To Common Problems

ome remedies have long endured a reputation in Western cultures of being helpful for only minor problems; on some level, many of us still undervalue their simple and powerful nature. For the majority of the world, though, home-remedies are the foundation of a healthy existence. And, in truth, caring for the mind and body, as well as the self and spirit at home would prevent many of the problems that plague us today.

Here, as elsewhere, it is helpful to employ the idea that, "less *is* more". Although we can fight disease with major weapons like specialists, hospitals, extreme therapies (such as chemotherapy), conventional medication, and radical surgery, we should first rely on ourselves and what nature makes available to prevent major health problems. Self-reliance will help us to avoid major crises that could impose the need for external intervention.

Given our planet's current state of disease, it is unrealistic to believe that these major ailments can be avoided completely. Practicing healthy natural living at home, however, can prevent many severe health problems.

Let us consider one of our major health problems— Cancer. Not only can we do a great deal at home to prevent cancer, we can also utilize many home remedies when facing it. The most important element in overpowering cancer is what we put, and, more importantly, do not put, into our bodies. The person who does not smoke, use drugs, or consume meat and dairy of any kind, including fish, milk, cheese, butter or eggs, but does exercise regularly, employ positive thinking, and engage his spiritual aspects avoids the cancers caused by severe abuses of living.

Many other common afflictions such as heart attacks, strokes and adult-onset diabetes (Type 2 Diabetes) can also be avoided by eliminating heavy, animal-based foods from the diet that obstruct our arteries and congest the cell's membrane.

You can control other problems, from teenage acne to Alzheimer's disease, with natural remedies and healthy living. The remedies listed here include nutrients, herbs, essential oils, therapies, and other forms of natural healing. These suggestions for prevention will not only help to accelerate healing, but may even make it unnecessary. All valid modern scientific research returns us to nature— the source of healing. And, today, there are a wide variety of natural therapies supported by credible scientific research. For example, Chinese researchers have found that the death rate from malaria, historically one of our world's most prevalent killers, can be significantly reduced with the traditional herbal medicine called, "artemisinin," while B-vitamins have been proven to avert heart attacks and severe birth defects, and even prevent broken bones as a result of osteoporosis.

Following is a suggested list of some health concerns and their at-home solutions (individual, chronic and/or extreme concerns require the counsel of a qualified practitioner):

DISORDER(S)	SOLUTION(S)
Abscesses	Chamomile; Slippery Elm; Zinc
Acne	Vitamin A; Vitamin E; Lecithin Vitamin B5 (Pantothenic Acid) Acidophilus; Chromium; Zinc Calendula; Echinacea; Goldenseal

ADDICTIONS:

Alcohol(ism)	B-vitamins; Vitamins D, E, K Probiotics; Magnesium; Thiamine Agrimony; Centaury; Cerato
Drug(s)	B-vitamins; Ginseng (for men) Gotu Kola (for women)
Tobacco (Smoking; Chewing)	B-vitamins; Vitamin C
AIDS (HIV)	Selenium; Zinc; Vitamin C Beta-Carotene; Vitamin B12 Olive-leaf Extract; Silymarin
Allergies (Dermatitis)	Essential Fatty Acids; Zinc B-vitamins; Vitamin E; Magnesium Bee-pollen; Burdock; Calcium Comfrey; Dandelion; Yerba Mate
Alzheimer's Disease (Senility)	Melatonin; Ginkgo Biloba; Anise B-vitamins; Vitamin E Supplemental oxygen
Amnesia (Memory Loss)	Ginkgo Biloba; B-vitamins Choline; Anise; Chromine Bee-pollen; Ginseng; Rosemary Blue-green Algae
Amyotrophic Lateral Sclerosis (ALS) (Lou Gehrig's Disease)	Calcium; Copper; Magnesium; Zinc, Vitamins B12, D, E

DISORDER(S)	SOLUTION(S)
Anemia	Folic Acid; Iron; Vitamin B12
Anxiety (Fear; Phobias; Tension; Depression; Melancholia; Stress; Seasonal Affective Disorder [SAD])	Aromatherapy; Massage-therapy Flaxseed-oil; Calcium B-vitamins; St. John's Wort Chamomile; Rose Hips Garlic; Selenium
Atherosclerosis	Vitamins A, C, E
Arthritis (Osteo-Rheumatoid)	Organic Sulfur; Kelp Nettle-leaf; Willow-bark Alfalfa; Calcium; B-vitamins Celery-seed Tea; Meadowsweet Parsley; Zingiber Offcinale
Asthma	Angelica; Bee-pollen Vitamins A, E; Yerba Mate
Athlete's Foot	Vitamin E; Garlic; Cone Flower Marigold; Myrrh
Attention Deficit Disorder (ADD; ADHD)	Choline; Essential Fatty Acids B-vitamins; Zinc; Ginkgo Biloba Ginger; Lemon Balm; Valerian
Autism	Magnesium Selenium; Zinc; Vitamins A, E
Autoimmune Diseases (Aging)	Beta-carotene; Vitamins A, E
Bacterial Infections	Grapefruit-seed Extract; Lapacho; Oregano-oil; Sarsaparilla-root
Bad Breath	Echinacea; Goldenseal; Parsley
Halitosis	Mint-oil; Vitamin C; Myrrh Rosemary

DISORDER(S)	SOLUTION(S)
Backache (Lumbago)	Vitamins A, E; Silicon Burdock; Horsetail; Slippery Elm
Bedsores	Goldenseal; Myrrh; Pau d'arco Vitamin E; Copper; Zinc
Bed Wetting	Buchu; Corn Silk; Oatstraw
Bites (Stings)	Vitamins C, E, Chamomile; Lavender; Echinacea, Elderflower; Red Clover
Blood-Pressure Problems	Cayenne; Celery; Chamomile
Hypertension	Fennel; Parsley; Vitamin E Calcium; Magnesium; Selenium
Body Odor	Fenugreek; Zinc
Boils	Goldenseal-powder; Parsley Slippery Elm; Burdock; Cleavers
Bone Spur(s)/Heel Spur(s)	Calcium; Magnesium; Chamomile; B-vitamins
Breast Health	Green tea; Melatonin; Turmeric Vitamins A, D, E; B-vitamins Calcium; Copper; Iodine; Zinc Magnesium; Selenium; Grapefruit
Bruises	Vitamin C; Comfrey-Poultice Witch Hazel; Alfalfa; Garlic

DISORDER(S)	SOLUTION(S)
Burns (Sunburn) (Skin Cancer)	Aloe Vera; Copper; Selenium; Vitamins A, C, E; Chamomile Elder Flower; Lavender; Zinc Marigold; St. John's Wort; Rosemary
Bursitis	Vitamins C, E Calcium and Magnesium
Cancer(s) **Melanoma** **Polyps**	Carotenoids; Feverfew; Garlic Ginger; Green Tea; Wheatgrass Vitamins A, C, D, E, K; B-vitamins Cabbage; Carrots; Cauliflower; Sprouts; Essential Fatty Acids Modified Citrus Pectin; Selenium, Raspberries; Strawberries; Algae; Zinc; Cesium
Canker (Cold-Sores)	B-vitamins; Vitamin E; Burdock Lysine
Carpal Tunnel Syndrome	B-vitamins; Calcium/Magnesium
Catarrh	Aromatherapy; Catmint; Chamomile; Elderflower; Eucalyptus; Hyssop
Chemical Poisoning	B-vitamins; Vitamin C Green Clay
Chicken Pox	Vitamins A, C; Silver Nitrate
Chlamydia	Vitamins C, E
Cholesterol (High)	Cayenne; Goldenseal; Kelp B-vitamins; Vitamin C Aloe Vera

DISORDER(S)	SOLUTION(S)
Chronic Fatigue Syndrome	Echinacea; Summa; Magnesium Essential Fatty Acids; Folate Vitamins A, C, E Acid
Circulatory problems (Chilblain)	Vitamin E; Zingiber Offcinale Elderflower; Lime-blossom Black Cohosh; Circu Formula
Cold(s) (Bronchitis)	Vitamin C; Osha; Garlic Lapacho; Zingiber Offcinale
Cold sores	B-vitamins; Lavender; Marigold
Fever blisters	Myrrh; Wild Indigo; Witch Hazel
Colic	Crushed Seeds of Caraway, Fennel or Marjoram; Peppermint Aniseed; Chamomile; Dill; Zingiber Officinale
Colitis	Vitamin E; Selenium; Garlic Flax-water; Aloe Vera
Constipation	Barley; Beans; Lentils; Peas Dandelion Root; Linseed Magnesium; Vitamins A, D
Cough(s)	Aromatherapy; Coltsfoot; Hyssop Thyme; White Horehound Vitamin C; Slippery Elm
Cramps	Cramp Bark (European Cranberry Bush); Zingiber Officinale; Vitamin E
Crohn's Disease	Essential Fatty Acids; Garlic Iron; Magnesium; Selenium; Zinc Aloe; Fenugreek; Probiotics

DISORDER(S)	SOLUTION(S)
Croup	Vitamin C; Fenugreek; Zinc
Cuts	Vitamin E; Comfrey; Marigold Myrrh; Witch Hazel
Cysts (Cystitis)	Vitamin E; Pure Water; Buchu; Chamomile; Meadowsweet
Cystic Fibrosis	B-vitamins; Vitamin C Echinacea; Goldenseal; Yarrow
Dandruff	B-vitamins; Vitamin E; Zinc Dandelion; Goldenseal; Kelp Hemp-seeds
Diabetes (I — II)	Essential Fatty Acids; Uva Ursa Fenugreek; Chlorella Vitamin C; Magnesium Chromium; Dandelion-root **AVOID SUGAR(S)!**
Diaper Rash	Vitamin E; Aloe-gel
Diarrhea	Apples; Bananas; Carrots; Garlic; Agrimony; Chamomile; Meadowsweet; Potassium; Vitamin E; Green Clay; Probiotics
Digestion Problems	Artichoke (leaves, extract) Black-radish juice Mint-oil; Vitamin K
Diverticulitis	B-vitamins; Cayenne; Chamomile; Garlic; Red Clover; Yarrow; Flax-water; Silver Nitrate; Probiotics

DISORDER(S)	SOLUTION(S)
Down Syndrome	Phosphatate; Blue-green Algae Chlorella; Vitamin B
Earache; Ear-Infection	Chamomile; Lavender; Manganese
Meniere's Syndrome (Ringing)	Vitamins A, C, E; Butcher's Broom; Supplemental Oxygen; Ginkgo Biloba
Eczema	Vitamin E; Zinc; Chickweed Comfrey; Heartsease; Marigold Nettle; Red Clover
Edema (Dropsy)	Vitamin B6; Dandelion; Garlic
Emphysema	Vitamin A; Magnesium; Rosemary
Endometriosis	Dong Quai; Summa; Vitamin E
Eye Problems: Cataracts	Vitamins A, C, E; B-vitamins; Zinc
Conjunctivitis; Glaucoma Photophobia; Xerophthalmia	Bioflavonoids; Melatonin; Garlic; Chamomile; Cayenne; Eyebright; Goldenseal Lutein (broccoli, kale, spinach)
Epilepsy	B-vitamins; Vitamin D; Lobelia Hyssop; Magnesium; Manganese
Fainting	Eucalyptus; Lavender Peppermint
Fatigue (Epstein-Barr Virus)	Magnesium; Iron; Potassium Acacia; Cayenne; B-vitamins Alphalipoic Acid; CoQ10

DISORDER(S)	SOLUTION(S)
Fever(s)	Water-Therapy; Elderflower Lobelia Extract; Vitamin A
Fibromyalgia (Muscle-Pain[s])	B-vitamins; Vitamin D; Melatonin; Cat's Claw Silver Nitrate
Flatulence	Anise; Catmint; Chamomile Lemon Balm; Probiotics
Fluid retention (Swelling Of The Ankles)	Geranium; Grapefruit; Juniper Lemon; Rosemary; Dandelion Leaf; Vitamin K; Potassium Supplemental Oxygen
Food poisoning (Salmonella)	Garlic; Potassium; Lobelia Aloe vera; Green Clay
Foot problems	Silica; Tiger Balm; Epsom-salt Footbaths
Fractures	Vitamins C, D; Zinc; Silica Calcium; Kelp; Magnesium
Frigidity	B-vitamins; Vitamin E; Kelp Bee-pollen; Summa; Gotu Kola
Fungal infections	Garlic-oil; Lapacho Fermented corn Extract Grapefruit-seed Extract
Gall bladder problems	Chamomile; Dandelion Root Fennel; Horsetail; Parsley Potassium; Hemp-seed
Gangrene (Dry, Wet)	Butcher's Broom; Echinacea
Glandular disorders	Dandelion; Echinacea; Parsley Vitamin A; B-vitamins; Zinc

DISORDER(S)	SOLUTION(S)
Gout	Vitamin C; B-vitamins Birch; Burdock-root; Cherries Celery Seed; Devil's Claw
Gynecological Problems	Vitamin E; Aloe Vera Primrose Oil; Wild-yam Creams
Hay Fever	Vitamins A, C; B-vitamins Chamomile; Eyebright; Ground Ivy; Ribwort
Headache(s) (Migraine[s])	Feverfew; Magnesium; Manganese; B-vitamins; Oxygen; Chamomile Lime-blossom; Peppermint Rosemary; Aromatherapy
Hearing impairment(s) (Tinnitus)	Vitamins A, C, D; B-Vitamins Ginkgo Biloba; Iodine; Iron; Magnesium; Zinc
Heartburn (Acidity)	Chamomile; Lemon Balm; Aloe Vera; Meadowsweet; Slippery Elm
Heart problems **Heart Disease** **Cardiovascular Disease** **Heart attack** (Myocardial Infarction)	Vitamins A, B1, B6, B12, C, D, E, K; Barberry; Dandelion; Summa; Beta Carotene; Chromium; Zinc; Folic Acid; Lycopene; Niacin; Magnesium; Potassium; Selenium
Hemophilia	Blue-green Algae Vitamin K; Wheatgrass
Hemorrhoids	Lemons; Oranges; Pure Water Dandelion; Goldenseal; Marigold Horse Chestnut; Milk Thistle; Nettle; Pilewort; Witch Hazel; Vitamins A, C; Rectal salve

DISORDER(S)

SOLUTION(S)

Hepatitis (A, B, C)	Selenium; Maitake Mushrooms Silver Nitrate; Milk Thistle
Hernia (Hiatal)	Comfrey; Goldenseal; Red Clover
Herpes (1 and 2)	Vitamins A, C, E; B-vitamins; Myrrh; Echinacea; Camphor
Hyperactivity	B-vitamins; Calcium; Magnesium; Fenugreek
Hypoglycemia (Low Blood Sugar)	Avocado; Chromium; B-Vitamins Fenugreek; Green Algae (chlorella) **AVOID SUGAR(S)!**
(post-)Hysterectomy	Calcium; Magnesium; Potassium B-vitamins; Vitamin C; Aloe Vera; Cat's Claw
Indigestion (Dyspepsia)	Gingerroot; Mint; Enzymes Chamomile; Meadowsweet; Papaya
Infection(s)	Vitamins A, C; Silver Nitrate Cranberry-seed-powder; Calcium Magnesium; Supplemental Oxygen
Infertility	Dong Quai; Gotu Kola; Zinc Vitamin E; Wild Yam extract Blue-green Algae
Inflammation (Chronic)	Nettle-leaf; Vitamins C, E, K Echinacea; Clover; Goldenseal; Pau d'arco

DISORDER(S)	SOLUTION(S)
Influenza (Flu)	Boneset; Echinacea; Garlic Melatonin; Lapacho Vitamins A, C; Slippery Elm Flaxseed Water
Immune System Problems	Echinacea; Pau d'arco; Pollens; Vitamins A, C, E, K Medicinal Mushrooms Green/Blue-green Algae
Impotence	Damiana; Oatstraw; Rosemary Ginseng; Gotu Kola; Vitamin E
Indigestion (Dyspepsia)	Chamomile; Fennel; Fenugreek
Intestinal Problems	Apples; Beans; Carrots; Peas Aloe Vera Juice; Probiotics Fenugreek-extract
Irritable Bowel Syndrome	Peppermint Oil/Caraway Oil Cascara Sagrada; Chamomile Lobelia; Pau d'arco; Rose Hips Probiotics; B-vitamins Vitamin E
Jaundice	B-vitamins; Vitamins C, E; Silymarin; Burdock; Fennel Echinacea; Green Tea; Thyme
Jet Lag	Melatonin; Supplemental Oxygen Eucalyptus-oil
Kidney Disease(s) (Stones) **Nephritis** (Bladder Problems)	Magnesium/Potassium; Calcium Iron; B-vitamins; Ginkgo Biloba Nettle; Parsley; Uva Ursa Pure Water (12 glasses per day)
Laryngitis	Agrimony; Sage; Thyme

DISORDER(S)	SOLUTION(S)
Lead Poisoning	Calcium; Magnesium; Garlic Vitamin C; Green Algae; Zinc
Learning Disabilities (ADD; Dyslexia; Hyperactivity)	Organic Lecithin Blue-green Algae; Hemp-seeds Green-sprout Juice
Leukemia; Lymphoma (Hodgkin's/non-Hodgkin's Disease)	Grass-juices; Vitamin A Medicinal Mushrooms; Green Tea; Pollens; Green/blue-green Algae; Cesium
Leukorrhea	Essential Fatty Acids; Garlic Pau d'arco
Liver-problems (Cirrhosis)	B-vitamins; Vitamins C, E Alfalfa; Silymarin Burdock; Fennel; Lemon Echinacea; Green Tea; Thyme
Lupus	Phenylalanine; Tyrosine Echinacea; Goldenseal Vitamins A, C; Alphalipoic Acid; CoQ10
Lyme Disease	Echinacea; Goldenseal; Summa Silver Nitrate; Cat's Claw
Macular Degeneration (Dry; Wet)	Ginkgo Biloba; Grapeseed-extract Wheatgrass juice
Malabsorption syndrome	Acidophilus; B-vitamins Aloe Vera; Soaked Flaxseeds
Malaria	Artemisinin
Manic-Depressive Disorder	Green/Blue-green Algae; Zinc B-vitamins; L-Tryptophan

DISORDER(S)	SOLUTION(S)
Measles	Chamomile; Elderflower Pau d'arco; Tea Tree Oil Lavender
Meningitis	B-vitamins; Phosphorous Horsetail; Frankincense
Menopausal Problems (Hot Flashes)	B-vitamins; Vitamin E; Sage Chaste Tree; Summa Wild yam-extract
Menstrual Irregularities (Pre-Menstrual Syndrome [PMS]) (Pre-Menstrual Symptoms)	Vitamins A, B6, C, D, E Calcium; Magnesium; Zinc Chamomile; Lemon Balm; Valerian; Cramp Bark (European CranberryBush); Lady's Mantle; Yarrow Chamomile; Chaste Tree; Cleavers
Mononucleosis	Dandelion; Echinacea; Goldenseal; Pau d'arco; Vitamins A, E; Silver Nitrate
Morning sickness	Chamomile; Zingiber Officinale Vitamin K; Supplemental Oxygen
Motion sickness	Magnesium; Zingiber Officinale (ginger); B-vitamins
Mouth, Teeth, Gums (Gingivitis) (Periodontal Disease)	Vitamins A, C, E Acid; Green Tea Folic Acid; Phytoplenolins Oregano Oil; Prickly-ash Bark; Selenium
Multiple Sclerosis (MS)	Vitamin C; Calcium; Thiamin Riboflavin; Potassium; Kelp Cat's Claw; Silver Nitrate Lemon-juice; Pollens

DISORDER(S)	SOLUTION(S)
Mumps	Vitamins A, C; Echinacea Rose Hips; Peppermint
Muscular Dystrophy	Vitamin E; Selenium Sea-Algae; Blue-green Algae
Muscle pain (Fibrositis; Cramps)	Vitamins A, E; Calcium; Magnesium; Meadowsweet; Willow Bark
Myasthenia Gravis	B-vitamins; Aloe Vera; Vitamins A, C, E; Manganese Skunk Cabbage
Myofascial Syndrome	Probiotics; Pure Water B-vitamins; Complete Minerals Trace Minerals
Nail-Problems	Biotin; Riboflavin; Iron; Zinc Calcium; Magnesium; Vitamin E Fermented-corn Extract; Silica
Nerve Problems (Neuropathy) (Neuralgia) (Neuritis) (Sciatica)	Essential Fatty Acids; Rosemary Vitamin E; Lavender; Chamomile Rosemary; Lime-blossom; Zinc Cramp Bark (European Cranberry Bush); Blue-green Algae
Nausea and Vomiting	Zingiber Officinale; Chamomile Vitamin D; Manganese
Nosebleed	Vitamin E; Yarrow; Witch Hazel
Obsessive-Compulsive Disorder	Green Tea; Blue-green Algae Enzymes

DISORDER(S)	SOLUTION(S)
Osteoporosis (Bone Loss)	Boron; Calcium; Magnesium; Zinc Silica; Silicon; Vitamin K; B-vitamins
Pain (Chronic; Acute)	B-vitamins; Vitamins C, E Boron; Magnesium; Clove Oil Feverfew; Ginger; Acupuncture Magnetic Therapy
Pancreatitis	Calcium; Magnesium; B-vitamins Hemp; Blue-green Algae
Parkinson's Disease	B-vitamins; Vitamin C; Pure Water; Sea/Fresh-water Algae
Phlebitis	Vitamins A, E, K; Capsicum Ginkgo Biloba
Pneumonia	Vitamins A, C; Silver Nitrate Eucalyptus Oil; Spearmint Oil Osha; Wintergreen
Poison Ivy/Poison Oak	Vitamins C, E; Camphor Echinacea; Goldenseal; Myrrh Rubbing Alcohol; Peroxide
Prostate Problems	Lycopene(s); Vitamin E; Zinc Boron; Selenium; Saw Palmetto Pygeum-extract; White Deadnettle
Psychological Problems	GABA Protein; Phytoleneline L-Tryptophan; Fresh-water Algae
Raynaud's Syndrome	Vitamins C, E; Garlic
Raynaud's Disease	Essential Fatty Acids; Cayenne

DISORDER(S)	SOLUTION(S)
Rheumatic Fever	Vitamin C; Garlic; Cat's Claw
Rheumatism	Dandelion; Nettle; Meadowsweet; Zingiber Officinale; B-vitamins
Ringworm (Parasites)	Vitamin E; Artemisinin; Paragon
Schizophrenia	Ginkgo Biloba; Algae Extracts Alpha Lupoic Acid; Tyrosine
Sexually transmitted diseases Candidiasis; Chlamydia; Herpes Genital Warts; Gonorrhea; Pelvic Inflammatory Disease (PID) Syphilis; Trichonomiasis Cervical Cancer (AIDS/HIV listed separately)	B-vitamins; Vitamin C; Kelp Probiotics; Garlic-oil; Zinc Echinacea; Goldenseal Silver Nitrate; Lemon-oil Medicinal Mushrooms; Pollens; Una da Gata
Shingles (Herpes Zoster)	Echinacea; Green-Tea Extract Lavender; Lime-Blossom; Oatstraw; B-vitamins; Vitamins C, D, E; Zinc; Supplemental oxygen
Sinus Problems	Garlic; Vitamins A, C
Sinusitis	Catmint; Elderflower Salt-flushes; Rose Water
Sjogren's Syndrome	Essential Fatty Acids; Zinc
Skin Problems (Moles, Psoriasis, Rashes, Ringworm, Seborrhea, Sores, Warts, Age-Spots, Vitiligo/Leukoderma)	Vitamins A, C, E; Aloe Vera Lecithin; Yellow Dock; Neem Cleavers; Dandelion-Root; Nettle B-vitamins; Oxygen
Scleroderma (Systemic Sclerosis)	Ointment

DISORDER(S)	SOLUTION(S)
Sleep Disorders (Insomnia)	Chamomile; Hyssop; Lemon Balm; Calcium; Magnesium; Lady Slipper; Lime-blossom; Jin Bu Hun; Passionflower; Valerian
Sore Throat (Tonsillitis)	Eucalyptus; Lemon; Agrimony; Chamomile; Echinacea; Myrrh; Pau d'arco; Sage; Thyme; Vitamins A, C; Tea Tree Oil
Spinal irregularities (Curvature; Disk Displacement; Pain; Posture; Scoliosis)	Comfrey; Wheatgrass; Silica Magnesium; Copper
Sprains and Strains	Comfrey; Marigold Tiger Balm-ointment
Stroke (Cerebral Aneurism)	Ginkgo Biloba; Magnesium Essential Fatty Acids; Choline Carrots; Pumpkins; Red Peppers
Sunburn	Vitamin E; Aloe Vera Flax/Hemp/Olive-oil
Temporomandibular Joint Syndrome (TMJ)	Hops; Passionflower; Valerian Calcium; Magnesium; B-vitamins
Thrombosis (Blood Clots)	Garlic; Ginkgo Biloba; Green Tea Essential Fatty Acids Grape-Juice; Nettle-Leaf
Thrush	Cone Flower; Marigold
Thyroid (para — hyper — hypo)	Iodine; Magnesium; Selenium Tyrosine; Cabbage; Cauliflower
Toxicity (Toxic Shock)	Calcium; Magnesium; Garlic; Zinc; Vitamins C, E; Kelp: Selenium; Green Clay

DISORDER(S)	SOLUTION(S)
Tuberculosis	Vitamins A, C, D, E; B-vitamins Selenium; Echinacea; Pau d'arco
Tumors (Benign; Malignant)	Barberry; Dandelion; Pau d'arco Red Clover; Vitamin C Fresh-water Algae; Grass-juices
Ulcers (Internal, Legs, etc.)	Vitamin E; Cabbage; Comfrey Tea Chamomile; Goldenseal; Myrrh Cayenne Pepper; Anti-Microbial Herbs
Urinary Problems (Incontinence; Infection)	Cranberry-Juice; Probiotics Horsetail; Pure Water
Varicose Veins	Horse Chestnut; Marigold; Potash Lime-Blossom; Witch Hazel; Vitamin C
Vertigo	Butcher's Broom; Cayenne Ginkgo Biloba; B-vitamins Vitamins C, E
Viruses	Vitamins C, E; Zinc; Echinacea; Pau d'arco; Silver Nitrate; Cat's Claw; Anti-microbial Herbs
Vision Impairment(s) (Glaucoma) (Retinopathy) (Cataracts)	Eyebright; Vitamins A, C; Zinc Magnesium; Selenium; Green Tea; Grass-juices
Weight (overweight; Underweight) (Obesity; Anorexia; Bulimia)	Avocado; Guarana; Stevia; Zinc Chromium; Magnesium Potassium; Selenium; Essential Fatty Acids; B-vitamins Chamomile; Myrrh; Green Algae; Dulse

DISORDER(S)	SOLUTION(S)
Whooping Cough	Chamomile; Coltsfoot; Lavender Thyme; White Horsehound Vitamins C, E; Cesium
Wound(s)	Aloe Vera; Copper; Zinc Vitamins B5, C, E; Hyperbarics Magnetic Therapy; Therapeutic Touch; Ultrasound
Yeast Infection(s) (Candida)	Biotin; Garlic; Goldenseal Vitamin C; Pau d'arco Oregano-oil; Olive-leaf Extract

All of these nutrients should be taken in their natural or food-based form. The fact that many of the solutions in this list are used for a *variety* of conditions indicates that the core of health and healing truly does exist in nature. Let us celebrate the bounties that she bestows upon us by honoring them in our daily life.

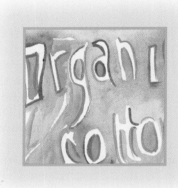

EIGHT

Our Clothing And Our Environment: What Is On Us And Around Us

HEALTHY SURROUNDINGS

O ur health is affected by everything with which we interact. These influences are far greater than we might consider and include everything from our clothing, our adornments, our homes, schools and workplaces, to our vehicles and other means of transportation. We must also consider the ways in which we construct, heat, cool, maintain and repair them as well as the resources we use in these processes. Other factors include the people, with whom we interact, our pets and recreations, as well as where and when we sleep and other forms of rest. The sensory impact of our environment is enormous, and extends beyond our primary communication methods of computers and cell phones, to what we 'take in' through our media and entertainment. Our health is so greatly affected by a vast number of external influences that it is critical to examine your life and make changes that will engage the basic aspects of living. Let us briefly discuss each of them:

MAN-MADE ENVIRONMENTS AND STIMULI

BUILDINGS

We spend more than 80% of our time indoors. It may surprise you to know that the average modern home contains 5-7 times more pollution than most major cities! Our workplaces— factories, offices or shops– and areas where we gather to dine, dance, watch sports, theater and movies, celebrate special events and attend conventions contain even more pollution than the average home. What we can control are our own spaces, so do what you can to make these areas as pollution free as possible by applying the following simple methods: 1. Use non-toxic materials for paint, carpeting, curtains, bedding, and other internal materials. 2. Ensure high quality air by cleaning your heating, cooling and filtering systems regularly and by providing for proper airflow and ventilation. 3. Dispose of all solvents, solutions, detergents, and cleansers that are not environmentally safe and health-friendly.

In areas where you cannot control the environment, choose to help yourself by gathering in places that do not permit smoking. The laws of many countries, states and communities now prohibit smoking in public places to ensure the health of both the smoker and non-smoker alike. Noise limitation and proper ventilation are, of course, very important for our hearing and breathing; avoid places with excessive noise and too little air. Also, use essential oils and oxygen, orally and internally, to reduce your chance of being infected in public places.

TRANSPORTATION

Most of us spend a large amount of time in automobiles, trucks, buses, trains, airplanes, boats and ships. People rarely walk and/or ride a bicycle for transportation; instead, we drive the shortest distances to do the simplest chores, increasing air-pollution as well as our weight. The materials inside our vehicles emit toxic, carcinogenic fumes, in addition to the poisonous fumes from the engine. Whenever you drive, even in the coldest of temperatures, open at least one window slightly to allow the carbon monoxide and other fumes to be released.

Buses, trains, monorails, railroads, and subways pose similar challenges, with an additional threat of contracting microbial infections from other passengers. When using rail transportation, you also face the dangers of electromagnetic field pollution inside and outside the passenger cabins.

Boats and ships also generate poisonous fumes that harm us as well as the life in our waters. If you are on water, you might need raw ginger or ginger-tea to settle your stomach and return your balance; they are among the best ways to calm seasickness.

Because of airtight cabins, the re-circulation of air, and very high levels of radiation, air transportation is very toxic; it is damaging not only to us, but also to our environment. Using oxygen and/or essential oils during your travels might help to deter any infections that you might catch on an airplane. And, wearing a polarizing device (a piece of jewelry, a card, or other magnetizing object) will help to divert harmful electrons from you, reducing the harmful effect of electromagnetic fields and radiation.

SLEEP AND OTHER FORMS OF REST

Next to proper food, clothing and shelter, restful sleep is the most significant aspect of a long and healthy life. Numerous scientific studies have proven the importance of sufficient rest, while confirming the many harmful effects of inadequate rest. Research conducted at Carnegie Mellon University and the University of Pennsylvania proved that a lack of sleep affects degrees of health, illness and even mucus production. Not surprisingly, people tend to sleep fitfully during serious illness; we stay awake for several hours, and then sleep for several more, repeating this cycle as the body battles to regain its natural rhythm. Sleep disruption, especially during sickness, is very unhealthy, and makes recovering from illness even more challenging. It is possible, for example, that many cases of the "24-hour flu" are the result of sleep deprivation rather than 'a bug'; and that the best prevention for a viral infection like the flu is proper, consistent sleep.

Sleep restores, renews and protects the cells of our immune system. Most of us need approximately eight hours of sleep per night; without it, not only is our quality of life compromised, but also our lives are shortened. The University of Buffalo published a study proving that sleep deprivation is cumulative. So, if you need eight hours of sleep per night but get only seven, by the end of a year, you will have lost 365 hours of life! Before the advent of artificial lighting, we lived on a dusk-to-dawn sleep pattern. Since the Industrial Revolution, however, the nightly sleep of Western Europeans and North Americans has declined from nine uninterrupted hours per night to seven often-interrupted hours. Those who are 18-54 sleep the least. After our 50s, the body requires the same amount of sleep, but often has less because of arthritic pain, stress, depression, various medications, and, for some, frequent nighttime trips to the bathroom.

As a result, many of us are out of touch with the natural rhythms of sleep and activity, especially those who work at night (appropriately called the 'graveyard shift'). These schedules not only affect our biorhythms, they interfere with our productivity and enjoyment of life. The ideal sleep pattern is to rest shortly after sundown and awaken shortly after sunrise. A brief, mid-day nap is natural, and a good addition to the usual eight hours of sleep per night. Unfortunately, our high-speed lifestyles, which include long commutes to and from work, preclude most of us from having a midday nap. During our senior years, however, it is necessary and natural to take many more naps during the day. Also, infants, children, teenagers, pregnant women, menopausal women, and those under unusual circumstances such as illness, grief or loss and other kinds of stress need more sleep than average.

We, at **Hippocrates Health Institute**, consider sleep, combined with positive attitude, raw living food, and regular proper exercise, essential to the best and healthiest life. In addition, our research has led us to revise our position about sleep medicines: if you have attempted legitimate natural sleep-aids without success, then apply Asian herbal medicine. If this natural medicine is still unsatisfactory, it is advisable to use prescription medicines—but responsibly and only temporarily— instead of battling constantly sleep loss, the results of which can be devastating.

Interestingly, we generally do not die from a physical disease; instead, we die either from sleep deprivation or from dehydration. Proper sleep increases your longevity, functioning, health, satisfaction and joy. And, every aspect of life depends on appropriate and consistent sleep. Most affected by lack of sleep are weight, diet, attitude and emotional levels, blood pressure and stress levels, as well as individuals at risk for heart disease and cancer. Even the capacity to reverse type-2 diabetes is significantly diminished by sleep deprivation.

First and foremost, disturbances in our sleep schedule create irregular and dangerous diets; lack of sleep causes cravings that we attempt to satisfy by eating cooked and processed carbohydrates, leading to such health problems as weight gain and altered brain chemistry. You can relieve these cravings by eating green vegetables and sprouts. You can also avoid sleeplessness by eating less or no fruit. **ALL FORMS OF SUGAR CAUSE SLEEP PROBLEMS!**

Keep in mind that vegetables have all the nutrients contained by fruits. So, they are the healthiest choice. It is important, though, to consider the amount of naturally occurring sugars in our vegetables and the effect they have on our blood sugar (commonly referred to as glycemic index.) Usually, foods grown underground, except in the onion family, are starchy and have more sugars. Because these foods have excess carbohydrates, eat them during winter when most vegetables, other than sprouts, are scarce. When food is grown above ground, with the exception of peas, corn and beans, it is low in starch and minimally glycemic.

In order to improve our sleep, nine-percent of us consume prescription drugs, four-percent take over-the-counter drugs, and three-percent use forms of alcohol. The National Sleep Foundation advises us to avoid alcohol as a sleep-aide because, although it is a sedative, it interrupts normal sleep patterns and interferes with our brain function. Research shows that when a person is intoxicated and then sleeps, their brain capacity and thinking ability are reduced by as much as 40% the following day! In addition to its many other benefits, **The Hippocrates Health Program** helps you to re-establish your normal sleep rhythms. Other types of rest such as meditation, prayer, yoga, and contemplation, which are offered at the Institute, are known to restore vitality and provide benefits equal to that of sleep. You can see discussions of these forms of rest in other publications from Hippocrates.

SENSORY INPUT

Take time to be aware of and regulate what you see, hear, touch, taste and smell, both in our natural and man-made environments and for yourself and your family. And, be careful not to put yourself into overload. Our complex technological age has presented many challenges, through such influences as the media and other forms of entertainment, that we must consciously and continuously work with to restore and maintain health.

SOUND(S): Shrill, high pitched artificially-generated sounds increase stress levels and decrease immunity. From Brahms to Broadway, pleasant, positively stimulating compositions have been shown to promote positive states of mind and overall health. These melodies should be part of your daily life. From the joyous gurgles of babies to the contented tones of our pets, sweet sounds not only constitute peaceful listening but they also relax the nervous system, thereby balancing – our bodies, minds, emotions and spirit, both individually and collectively.

SIGHTS: Dark, dreary surroundings drain the spirit and lead to fear and depression. Surround yourself with only positive, attractive visual input, whether natural, artistic or technical and you will notice an enormous difference in how you feel. The light that enters your iris stimulates brain chemistry and plays a major part in your emotional moods by generating balance and harmony. Negative visual stimulation causes the opposite response; it increases stress, insecurity and negative moods. Since what we see affects who we are and how we respond to life, we must not only choose but also create and recreate environments that provide us with positive visual images that reflect a positive world. Be selective in everything that you and your family see, hear, touch, taste, and smell and you will reap great rewards!

WHAT WE TOUCH: Loving touch is basic to all of life; unwarranted and unwanted touch is a terribly isolating experience, the repercussions of which are often felt for a lifetime. If all touching were constructive, as it should be, it follows that all of our efforts would be constructive as well. Therapeutic massage, for example, is a formal means of promoting health on all levels. Science has proven that healing touch is of direct, immediate, substantial and permanent benefit to all forms of life. Researchers at the

University of Miami have conducted studies to verify the beneficial impact of positive touch on infants— tender touch increases immunity.

Nature has provided us with many glorious sensory experiences: the feeling of a flower against your fingers; the sensation of walking in the sand; the flowing caress of warm ocean water; and, the softness of your pet's hair. These joyous interactions, and many others like them, confirm our union with nature. We are truly 'touched' when we allow ourselves this communion from a place of reverence, respect and gratitude.

WHAT WE TASTE: Just as nature provides an abundance of experiences to hear, see and touch, it also endows us with a banquet of delicacies to taste. This banquet of foods, the cornerstone of **The Hippocrates Living-Foods Program**, is an essential element of health—one that we teach extensively at the Institute and one we must protect and nurture with tremendous resolve. It is no secret that like many other things in our lives, our food supply is very polluted. There are many volumes that are offered through the Institute's store that speak of this great challenge. It is time now for all of us to spread the word to the people we care about that much of what we take into our body is the cause of great pain. As we elevate ourselves and our world by living healthfully, we will refine both our creation and appreciation of this superb bounty of nature.

"THE NOSE KNOWS:" During this age of rampant pollution, we experience an entire range of odors from fragrant to foul. Every aroma generates both psychological and physical sensations and consequences. Fine fragrances benefit both your psyche and your system, but airborne germs and bacteria can create an intolerable stench that causes headaches, watery eyes, and other irritations of both body and spirit. Sadly, many have also violated the respiratory tract with a variety of 'drugs,' from over-the-counter inhalers to cocaine. Our noses have highly sensitive membranes. As such, it is critical to honor them, using only healthy substances prescribed by qualified, expert practitioners.

Delightful fragrances, such as essential oils, are wonderful for the home and the workplace; they intensify your senses and increase the neuronal activity in your brain. Many scientific studies have also proven that these pleasant aromatics elevate comprehension and intensify creativity.

POWDERS, PERFUMES, COSMETICS AND OTHER PENETRATING PREPARATIONS: PROBLEMS

While we benefit significantly from the pleasant and positive natural preparations that we put into and onto our bodies, we also suffer from the toxic effects of synthetic ones. To promote health, select organic products that nourish your skin and spirit, rather than petroleum-based, chemically formulated concoctions. Natural mineral-based makeup, perfumes and lotions are readily available worldwide. These botanical creations nourish you and your skin, keeping you fresh and healthy; and, typically, you will not need as much of a natural product to achieve even more pleasing results.

TOILETRIES— toothpaste, mouthwash, and deodorant to name a few— are critical both to your health and hygiene. Conventional toothpastes and mouthwashes often contain fluoride, alcohol, foaming agents derived from petroleum products, or dyes, all of which are permanently destructive not only to teeth and gums but to your entire system. Commercial deodorants often contain aluminum, which is toxic and irritating to your skin and weakens your immune system. Also, commercial perfumes and colognes are laden with formaldehydes and other poisonous chemicals. So, instead of eliminating disease-causing microbes, these poisonous products force your body to defend itself against them!

Discovering these fine contributions to your health and beauty is incredibly rewarding. The Internet is a wonderful resource; however, frequenting stores and boutiques that feature these luxurious products is a pampering and beautifying experience in itself. The purest plant-based solutions (in both "senses" of the word) are also available from **The Hippocrates Health Institute** gift store, which you can visit online, by phone or in person.

One final consideration: all commercial products are tested on helpless and innocent animals— most which suffer immeasurable pain and eventual death to ensure the 'safety' of a product for human consumption. It is unquestionably worthy and life giving to support companies who are opposed to the use of animal products and testing of any kind; you will find a wide variety of these products in health food stores and specialty stores. It is an absolute truth that when we revere life on all levels, our bodies, minds and spirits soar.

INGESTING DISASTER

CHEMICAL SUPPLEMENTS— man-made and chemically contrived vitamins, minerals, proteins, "low-fat" and "low-carb" creations, hormones, steroids, and drugs (medicinal and "recreational") — are harmful because they can cause permanent debility and even death.

As a society, we are ingesting these artificial concoctions at alarming rates. Amazingly, many of the manufacturers of these synthetic supplements claim them to be "natural!" The fact is that more than 90% of man-made supplements are not from truly natural sources! The remaining relatively modest percentage of supplementation is based upon whole food. When choosing supplements for your family, select only whole food supplements, as artificial supplements damage the immune system and cause disease, premature aging, and other severe physical, psychological and emotional difficulties. We face another very difficult challenge with international multi-billion-dollar pharmaceutical companies, who are successfully generating an ever growing and misinformed, consumer base. The pharmaceutical industry is intent upon controlling the supply of supplements, and is already perilously close to doing so. In Europe, for example, many supplements can be acquired only by prescription. The inadequacy of products aside, the consequences of this international conspiracy are obvious and severe: monopolization leads to indecent pricing.

Food-based supplements, on the other hand, build your health naturally. And, because they are natural, they cause no adverse effects. Pollens, algae, whole-food-based vitamins, minerals and proteins, and other such organic selections benefit your immune system, stabilize hormonal activity, provide oxygen, initiate and maintain chemical balance, and increase enzyme function. In my work both at **Brandal** and at **Hippocrates**, I have found whole-food supplements beneficial both to the healthy and the healing.

"Low-fat" and "low-carb" concoctions, like the many such fad diets they support, are dangerous and destructive. In theory, "low-fat" and "low-carb" "foods" are useful; however, because they are commercially processed, they disturb your metabolism and rob you of nutrients, thereby depleting your enthusiasm, vitality and focus. Even your ability to rest and sleep is compromised when consuming fabricated foods. These popular but often dangerous 'diets' are the result of misinformation and unrestrained economic manipulation. The combination of a living-food diet, proper exercise, and positive living is the best way to create, secure and maintain complete health, and full function, including your desired weight.

Man-made hormones are also notorious for causing permanent damage. HRT (Hormone Replacement Therapy) has been implicated in various diseases. In my work, I have encountered many women who developed cancer as a result of this "therapy." I have also witnessed cardiovascular issues and liver malfunction due to the irresponsible and extensive use of artificial, hormone-based, so called "thyroid medicines."

Birth control pills and devices also create various problems for many women. The prolonged use of birth control pills has been implicated in instances of early menopause, liver disorders, and even the obstruction of capillaries. Devices such as IUDs are irritants that scrape uterine walls, causing painful, permanent scarring, fibroid tumors and cysts, and possibly even cancer.

While early menopause plagues many middle-aged women, early menstruation plagues many young girls. During and before the early Twentieth Century, average menstruation began in the mid to late teens. Today, it often commences at pre-teen ages! These drastic interruptions of the joys of girlhood are a result of chemical saturation caused by polluted water, food, air, clothing, and an essentially polluted environment. We must recognize that our way of living is causing a radical restructuring of natural law; early menstruation and early menopause not only robs women of their due childhood, but also robs them of their deserved maturity.

SYNTHETIC HGH— Human Growth Hormones— and other hormonal products such as DHEA, and man-made testosterone, progesterone, and estrogens are causing great concern among consumers and the health community alike. "Chemists" of limited ability with unlimited ambition are manufacturing products from their laboratories without regard for their total safety. There are, however, some legitimate manufacturers who are providing homeopathic versions of these hormones, which can greatly enhance the body's function.

Steroids, used by both patients and athletes, and prescribed by practical physicians as well as dubious "doctors," have become a severe health hazard. Excessive use of steroids either as medicine or as artificial bodybuilding aides eventually causes all of the body's vital organs to fail, resulting in permanent damage and the hastening of death. Although legitimate steroids have benefits when properly used, many are overused, misused and abused with catastrophic consequences.

The regular use of steroids to enhance athletic performance results in an intense alteration of brain chemistry, heart malfunction, abnormal growth patterns, muscle degeneration, body deformity, premature aging, and untimely death. As a society, we are abnormally fixated on winning, so much so that we not only violate natural laws, but also our bodies, our health, our development, and our very future as a viable life form. It is crucial for each one of us to see where we may be compromising our health for the sake of winning or looking good, so we can return to nature and reverse these severe effects.

Other types of drugs, both medicinal and "recreational," are destroying many lives and families. Multinational pharmaceutical companies are more controlling than ever, putting profit before people and money before morality. Those of us who are plagued by fear and such problems as low self esteem tend toward addiction and often turn to drugs for escape. Drugs erode our spirit and our humanity. Self destructive addictions to everything from tobacco, food and alcohol to pain-killers, cocaine and other abused prescription drugs like OxyContin turn many of us into burdens—to our families, our communities and our world. We sacrifice the absolute reality of responsibility for the fleeting illusion of security. Even the habitual use of marijuana, which is medically prescribed and even socially accepted in some areas of the world, dramatically increases our vulnerability to cancer. Either occasional or chronic abuse of marijuana also causes diminished mental capacity, which often precipitates senility.

Medicine has been of great benefit to us. However, when it is used excessively or inappropriately, whether for short or long periods, it betrays and brutalizes. Medicine was intended to benefit and build, as clearly supported by the Hippocratic Oath to which each and every doctor subscribes. 'First do no harm,' is a motto, that when followed and respected, will build health.

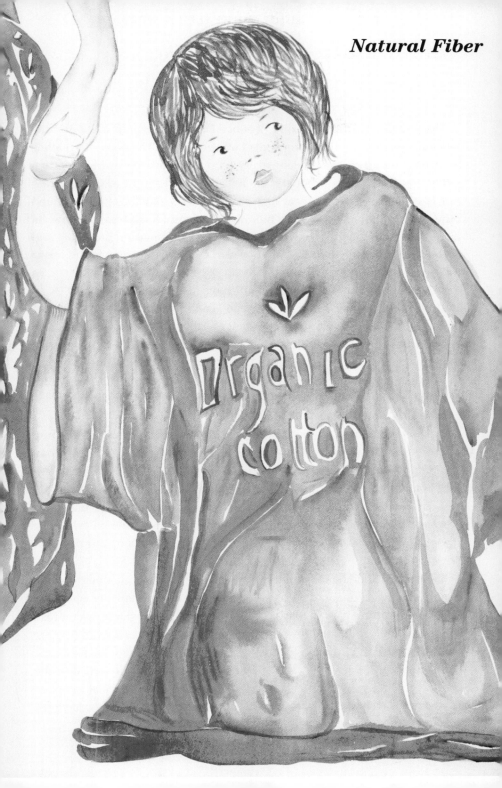

YOUR INTIMATE ENVIRONMENT

CLOTHING

Organically grown, naturally produced clothing is important for the health of your family. Our skin is the largest organ of the body; it breathes and absorbs and removes waste every second. As proven by the nicotine-patch and other such products, chemicals placed on the skin penetrate our bodies. So, when we wear man-made fibers — such as polyester and other 'microfibers' — the skin literally inhales their oil-based toxins. In most cases, body odor increases because the skin's natural breathing and detoxification process is choked; they also constrict movement and cause fatigue. In addition, the manufacturing of man-made fibers increases ecological pollution, causing even more disease and waste.

Cotton, flax, linen, hemp, tencel, and "compassionate" wool are some of the best materials for clothing; they are helpful to your skin and the environment. Organic cotton is especially ecological, as the production of non-organic cotton spreads 25% of the world's pesticides! There is a profound positive benefit to your health and spirit when you choose better clothing and wear other natural kinds of clothing such as shoes, socks, gloves, hats, and scarves.

It is encouraging to know that organic clothing is being used more and more, at a rate that exceeds 15-20% percent per year. Even the renowned "fashion-designer," Giorgio Armani has declared that, "it is possible to live with both style and awareness." Garments that benefit both body and ecology have sometimes been misperceived as earthy and extremely unstylish; however, modern designs are proving otherwise. Now, we can fulfill our responsibility to nature and to ourselves while also satisfying our desire to dress fashionably.

Comfortable and healthy undergarments are essential; purchase organic underclothing before anything else. Most men have a relatively easy time finding comfortable natural briefs, jockey-shorts and undershirts; by contrast, we as women are plagued by the prevalence of undergarments (except panties) that contain disease-causing chemically laden fibers. Research conducted by Sidney Ross Singer and Soma Grismaijer proved that the material content and styles of modern brassieres could cause cancer. Their study, called the "Bra and Breast Cancer Study (BBCS)," was conducted to assess the attitudes, values and behaviors of women about their breasts and brassieres. Sadly, this and other research support that both attitudes toward our bodies as well as our clothing have potential cancer-causing affects.

Furthermore, studies have shown that men who wear tight underwear are subject to testicular constriction that inhibits blood flow, causing low sperm count, impotence, and erectile dysfunction.

The intimate garments of babies and children are subject to cancer-causing, fire-retardant chemicals. Fortunately, however, clothing for children of all ages is readily available in organic, non-toxic, non-flammable forms.

BEDDING

It is evening. You remove both your outer garments and your undergarments, and you prepare for a restful sleep. You sleep either, "au natural," or you wear healthy organic natural pajamas. But, then, you climb into a bed that is not only disrupting your slumber but also compromising your health. What should have been your greatest comfort is, instead, a brief and bothered experience.

The bed can be full of toxic materials: metal springs in conventional mattresses attract renegade electric frequencies, cause cross-circuitry throughout your body and restrict the functioning of your immune cells, and synthetic, man-made fibers that constitute most mattresses pollute your bedroom, body and brain. Even modern mattresses that are made to conform to your body are made of toxic materials. So, while they might comfort you temporarily, they may irritate you permanently. Pillows are often filled with foam made of synthetics— so if you sleep on your stomach you literally encountering a face full of toxins! Pillows filled with feathers from birds that have suffered, not only hurt them but also you and your family by providing inadequate support for heads, necks and upper backs.

The best choices for maximum rest and foremost health are organic cotton-filled futons and natural airbeds covered with a thin organic mattress. Additionally, either organic cotton-filled or buckwheat-seed-filled pillows give us the best and healthiest sleep. Organic pillowcases, sheets and bed-covers provide the only means of healthy, comfortable, restful slumber. From flannel to Egyptian cotton, natural choices are the only safe ones.

CONCLUSION

As we can see, our environment— from inner to outer— not only comprises who we are, but how we function and interact in our world. It is a skill to create environments that are both functional and healthy. The Asians have known this for centuries, providing us with the art of **Feng Shui,** the arrangement of spiritually fulfilling and beautifully appropriate spaces. Feng Shui works with nature's elements, including color and form as well as the placement of furniture, plants and other physical aspects of our homes and workplaces. When you walk through a properly manicured home or botanical garden, you have a sense of peace and a feeling of unity. These natural spaces are structured to be in harmony with nature, respecting both its independence from and its interaction with us. Natural sounds, such as gentle pearls of water flowing into earthly basins, and harmonious beams of light, both natural and man-made, create a secure and profound sense of serenity and harmony.

Imagine interacting with healthy and joyous people in a complete, pure and harmonious environment…and then make it your reality, one step at a time!

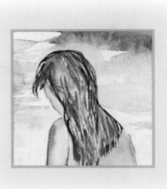

NINE

Baths, Thermal And Oxygen Therapies

During our exploration of environments, we uncovered the joy and healing of bathing. Today, many people are fortunate enough to prepare not only cleansing but also health promoting baths for themselves and their families at home or to travel short distances to enjoy specialized types of baths.

One of the easiest at-home baths is an aromatherapy bath; simply put six drops of selected essential oils on the surface of the bath water. These drops become a thin layer of healing that is partially absorbed into the skin. Among the conditions that are soothed by aromatherapy baths are arthritis, eczema, psoriasis, burns, bruises, emotional distress, viruses, bacteria, cancer, stress, fatigue, colds and flu, varicose veins, acne, premature aging, dehydrated skin, and detoxification.

Temperature-raising water therapies such as ginger baths help to break fevers and fight viruses and bacteria. Also, whirlpools pump and cleanse the lymphatic system, relax the nerves, and purify the bloodstream. Thousands have used these methods at The Institute and then at home to heal themselves. Following is a list of some of the most effective baths, natural water and thermal treatments and other stimulating therapies.

BODY-BASED THERAPIES

Soaking in pure water that has been enriched by organic oils or herbs has always been a fine way of healing and relaxation.

BATHS AND NATURAL WATERS

Artesian well-water Baths In many parts of the world, people drink water from Artesian wells. That is not advisable; however, soaking in this water stimulates the body's electrical system, allowing energy to flow freely through the meridians. These kinds of baths combine relaxation and healing.

Baking-Soda Baths One pound (1/2 kilogram) of baking soda (make sure that the baking soda is aluminum-free) dissolved in pure water in a standard bathtub is an excellent means of expelling heavy metals, radioactivity and chemical toxicity from the cells and tissues of your body.

Clove-Oil Baths Forty drops of pure clove oil placed into a warm bath helps to limit skin irritations that cause rashes and itching.

Dandelion-Extract Baths During spring and autumn, collect fresh whole dandelions — including the roots. Add their juices to your bath — approximately 1 quart (15 milliliters) for each warm tubful; soak for 20-30 minutes. This process helps to extract toxins, heavy metals and radiation from your skin and other organs.

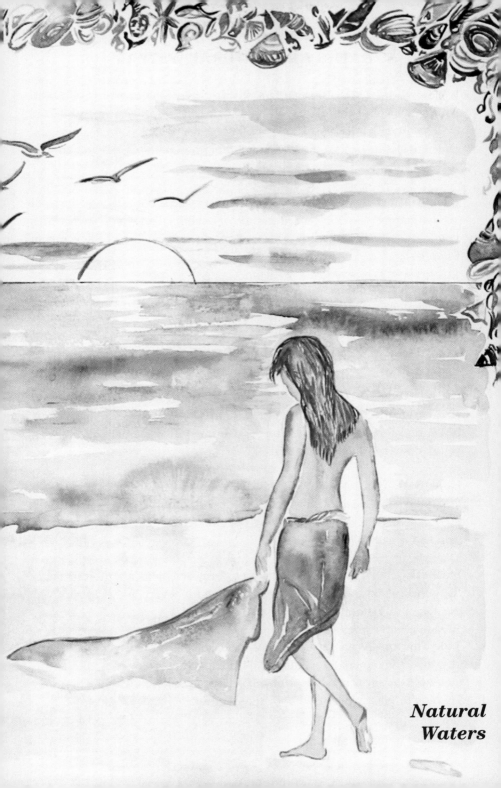

Natural
Waters

BATHS AND NATURAL WATERS

Epsom Salts (Sitz Baths) This form of hydrotherapy is effective to counteract skin eruptions such as eczema and psoriasis, many rashes, cystitis, hemorrhoids, prostate problems, muscle aches and spasms, and neurological disorders. Sit for a minimum of 45 minutes, up to 1 hour in luke warm water.

Essential-oil Baths Bathing in essential oils (the immersion form of aromatherapy) — with their multitude of beneficial effects — invigorates your skin, senses and spirit. Please see the extensive list of these oils in Chapter Six.

Fenugreek Infusions Juice 1/2 pound (1/4 kilo) of 7-day-grown fenugreek-sprouts; pour a small amount on a dry brush or hard-bristled natural brush; with circular motions, rub the brush against your skin in the areas of your liver, pancreas and gall bladder for no more than ten minutes; allow the juice to soak through your skin for 30 minutes before bathing.

Ginger-Bath 1/2 cup of pure ginger-powder dissolved in pure water in a standard bathtub enables you — gently, yet powerfully — to elevate your body temperature, thus helping to eliminate viruses, toxins, and other disease-causing life forms.

Hops-Bath Boil 1/4 pound (1/8 kilo) of bio/organic dried hops for 20 minutes; pour the fluid into your tub filled with hot water; soak in it for 30 minutes. This bath is not only relaxing but also soothing hydration for your skin and spirit.

Ice-Bath Unlike the warm therapeutic baths, ice baths are used to cause the pores to contract to eliminate waste and for severe burns, either from the sun or any other source.

Jade Therapy Asians have known the value of jade in healing for thousands of years. One ounce (30 milliliters) of jade powder added to a full hot tub increases energy (chi). Jade is also used in combination with Far Infrared Therapy to create increased body temperature.

BATHS AND NATURAL WATERS

Kelp-Baths Mix 4-8 ounces (120-240 milliliters) of kelp, and/or other types of seaweed, into a hot bath to improve skin texture, mineralize the body, and remove radioactivity and harmful acids.

Loofah-Sponge Baths The slightly rough texture of this natural sponge stimulates the removal of dead skin and external toxins while increasing circulation.

Mikvah Ceremonial immersion that combines physical and spiritual cleansing. Many devotees of the Sabbath and other traditions take these baths the day before the Sabbath. Baptism developed from this practice.

Mineral Water from Natural Springs Healing, natural water resorts exist throughout the world. Minerals are essential to the healing effect of all natural-spring baths. Most notable among them are sulphur-springs, which are famous for healing arthritic and osteoporotic disorders. Other minerals contained in these waters — depending upon their composition, quality and quantity — provide medicinal and soothing effects. Please note that — even today — there are undisturbed natural waters throughout the world; find them and enjoy them!

Noni-Juice Scrubs Mix 2 oz. (60 milliliters) of noni juice with 2 oz. of green clay. Then rub into the lymph glands of the neck and on the throat, and use as a facemask for hydration and healing.

Oil-of-Hemp Rub Hemp oil contains the most balanced and effective fatty acids that are necessary for healthy cell development. Rub this oil into areas of dryness, and spread it lightly on the body, including the face. Do this before sleep to allow the oil to soak through your body overnight. Place towels over your sheets for that night's sleep.

Powdered Lavender Apply lavender powder to all parts of the body after bathing to calm nerves, relieve stress, and induce rest.

BATHS AND NATURAL WATERS

Quinine-Baths Place 16 ounces (1/2 liter) of quinine water into warm bath-water; soak for 20-30 minutes. This process opens the capillaries, aids the respiratory system, and soothes all of the organs and the nervous system.

Raspberry-Seed Powder Mix 1 oz. (30 milliliters) of raspberry-seed powder with 1 oz. of pure water; mix into a paste; apply on temples and forehead, and allow to remain for a minimum of one hour. Stimulates neuron activity in the brain; useful against ADD, depression, and dyslexia.

Sea-Salt Baths Ocean water — because of its chemical likeness to human blood — enhances the benefits that you can derive from bathing in natural sea-water or sea-salt baths. Because of their exceptional mineral content, the Dead Sea and the Great Salt Lake are the most well known bodies of water for their curative powers. Bathing in water containing 5-8 cups of dissolved pure sea-salt in a standard bathtub benefits circulation, neurological function, healthy skin, detoxification, and overall relaxation.

Turkish-bath/Russian-bath/Steambaths The thermal water vapor that heats your body and enters your lungs gently elevates body temperature at the same time that it stimulates renal (kidney) and respiratory function, thus eliminating toxins and stress. The water based organs of the human body are strengthened by consistent use of the various types of steam baths.

Ultimate Detoxification On fasting days — while you are consuming wheatgrass juice, green juice and plenty of pure water — start the day with a self-administered deep massage using your hands and other massage equipment. Then, take a whirlpool-Jacuzzi or Epsom salt bath, soaking for 15-30 minutes. Then, rest in contemplation for one hour. Next, use a sauna, steam bath or ginger bath for 15 minutes to raise your body temperature. Pat yourself with a dry towel; place two towels on your bed; wrap yourself in towels, and cover yourself, preparing for rest that might include sleep.

Vinegar-Rubs Apply vinegar to every part of the body (add essential oils to neutralize the aroma.) This rub alkalizes the skin and bloodstream, ridding it of fat-based toxins.

BATHS AND NATURAL WATERS

Whirlpools/Jacuzzi Circulated and heated water under significant pressure assists the lymphatic system and other organs to release toxins. The neurological and muscular systems are stimulated, thereby releasing tension and lactic acids. These baths significantly minimize problems of the lymphatic system, the liver and the gall bladder.

Xanthium-Baths Juice 4 ounces (120 milliliters), and place into a full tub of hot water. Soak for 30 minutes. Relieves nausea, vomiting and dizziness.

Yucca-Root Therapy Cut a one-inch (2.54 centimeter) whole round piece of yucca; place it on pimples, open cysts, acne-blemishes, and other skin irritations. Leave for 15 minutes, 2-3 times per day. Helps to neutralize infection and heal and soften skin.

Zingiber Officinale (Jamaican Ginger) Tincture Press 1 ounce (30 milliliters) of this root; mix with 1 ounce of fresh lemon juice; leave for 2 hours. Then, place tincture on the veins of the forearms, back of the neck, and both temples. Leave to soak for several hours. Stimulates brain activity; removes mercury from the bloodstream and calms the digestive system.

Dry-Brushing Bristles of natural materials moved in a round clockwise motion (starting from the heart) on all parts of your body will remove the approximately 2 pounds (1 kilo) of waste that evaporate from your skin daily. Stimulation of the bloodstream and relaxation of all membranes are just some of the beneficial results of this pleasant process. Dry brushing is often used in combination with sauna and/or steam baths.

Dry Sauna Dry saunas utilize convection currents to warm you from the outside-in, raising body temperature; this beneficial process facilitates the elimination of microbes and mutagens from your system. Correct use of dry sauna assists detoxification. This type of sauna also has a healing effect on oil-based organs such as the liver and gall bladder. Dry sauna also helps to melt cholesterol and plaque in your veins.

BATHS AND NATURAL WATERS

Far Infrared Sauna (Long waves) This inside-out temperature-increasing therapy is used extensively against microbes and mutagens. Its electro-magnetic spectrum is divided into three segments by wavelengths. It produces significantly cooler air temperatures than the dry sauna because of its low energy band (from 7-14 microns). Far Infrared Sauna penetrates the tissues of the body deeply, releasing more perspiration and poison using a lower surface temperature than dry saunas. This allows you to spend more time in the sauna. Properly used as part of an effective natural health program, Far Infrared Sauna has 3 1/2 times the detoxifying effect than through general use.

Kneipp Therapy Father Kneipp formally introduced contact-with-nature-therapies. A significant part of Kneipp Therapy includes walking barefoot in the morning dew, in brooks and streams, and on river-rocks. Other therapies utilize herbs in hydrotherapy.

Sound-Therapy Everything from the gently wafting sounds of nature to the scientifically created electronic sounds of the Monroe Institute plays an important role in our psychological and physiological health. Many detailed studies have proven that harmonious sound elevates the positive hormones such as serotonin, increasing intellectual, emotional, creative and spiritual levels. For example, many cities play the recorded works of Mozart publicly, yielding positive, calming results. In his books, ***The Mozart Effect***, and, ***The Mozart Effect for Children***, Don Campbell, a music-healing educator, states that the director of Baltimore Hospital's Coronary Care Unit has said that 1/2 hour of classical music has the same benefit as 10 mg. of Valium! Mr. Campbell also reveals that students who sing and/or play a musical instrument score as much as 51 points higher on the SAT examination ("Scholastic Aptitude Test," given to American students in mathematics and language) than the national average!

OXYGEN-THERAPY (HYPERBARICS)

Hyperbarics is a modern method of using oxygen to improve ones health. There are two types of **Hyperbaric Therapy**, high-pressure and low-pressure. We, at **The Institute**, use the low-pressure method exclusively, because it has proven to be more effective in addressing the following ailments, among many others: bacterial infections, the effects of stroke, Lyme's Disease, hypoxia, Multiple Sclerosis, cerebral palsy, diabetic wounds, traumatic brain injuries, post-operative care, anti-aging, and loss of mental and physical energy.

Hyperbaric Therapy uses atmospheric pressure to provide more oxygen to the blood cells, blood plasma, cerebral spinal fluid, and all of the body. The Hyperbaric Chamber, in which this therapy is administered, supplies oxygen to affected areas, as well as supplemental oxygen when necessary for greater effectiveness.

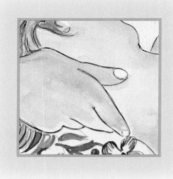

TEN

Body Therapies And Massage

W hatever your age, your body requires massage. From the beginning of time, harmonious contact among all creatures has enriched lives, the most intimate of which is touch. Each of us requires constant loving physical contact, the exchange of which elevates and energizes the functioning of every system, as proven in extensive research at the University of Miami. Although styles of touch are unique to individual cultures, appropriate therapeutic touch itself, and its many benefits, is universal. Individual forms of touch from many cultures created unique kinds of massage and bodywork.

The loving, supportive application of hands to the body begins at birth. The caring pediatrician, midwife, or family member that delivers the newborn handles her welcomingly. Then, she is given to the doting mother and father and the rest of the loving family, whose thrilled hands convey that they are loved and welcomed, a profound and positive memory that is with her for life. As the child grows, ever-loving, appropriate touches from parents, siblings, other family members, friends and pets continue the cycle of positive contact. The importance of touch to emotional and spiritual health is also received formally through massage, which is both enjoyable and beneficial to a person on all levels.

Massage is defined as the use of the hands to stimulate or soothe the soft tissues of the body for therapeutic purposes. While massage is useful for easing pain, reducing stress and relieving discomfort, it is also helpful in renewing and maintaining mental, emotional and even spiritual balance. Massage induces physical relaxation, promotes health and increases resistance to disease; it also increases flexibility and range of motion, reduces inflammation, increases the mobility of joints, improves muscletone and circulation, and relieves problems of nerves and muscles. Massage also helps to rest the body, not only during activity but also when you sleep.

The application of pressure eases the tension in the muscles, enabling the fibers to stretch and relax. This allows the blood to flow freely, releasing poisons both from the blood stream and from the rest of the body. The increased circulation also allows greater flow of oxygen and other nutrients to the affected areas. So, massage elevates the body's resistance to illness, disease and aging, leading to a longer, healthier and more energetic life.

MASSAGE IS NOT A LUXURY —
IT IS A NECESSITY!

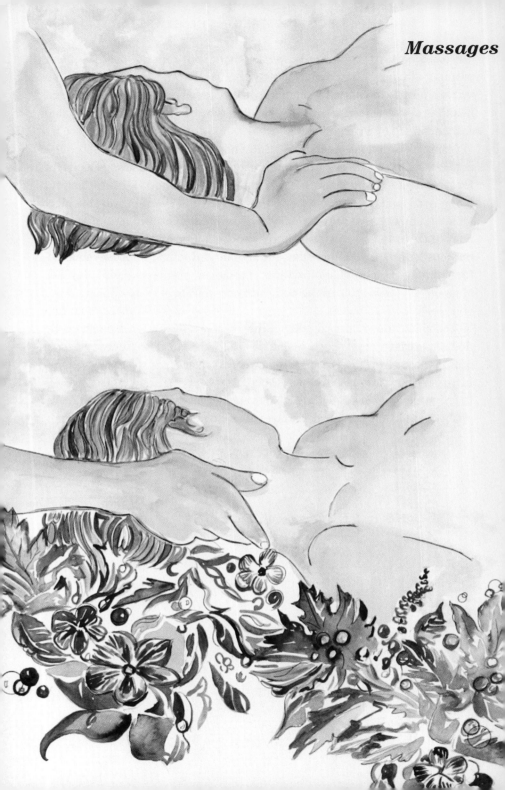

There are many types of massage. We will now discuss the ones most often used at **Hippocrates Health Institute** and most useful at home; this does not mean that other types of massage would not be of great benefit to you and your family. Massage affects everyone individually. But, all good massage must always feel safe, positive and non-invasive. Massage provides long range benefits, especially when enjoyed regularly. Following is a list of some of the most popular types of body-therapies and massage:

ACUPRESSURE

The specialized massage called, "acupressure," or, "ear acupressure," will be discussed in the next chapter in conjunction with the procedure called, "ear pressure".

CELLULITE MASSAGE

The application of special oils is designed to remove the undesirable and unsightly toxic deposits around the hips, thighs, and other areas of the body that accumulate cellulite. Daily treatments for a week have excellent results.

CRANIO-SACRAL THERAPY

This mode of massage is a gentle, non-invasive alignment of the body; it improves brain and spinal cord function. An adjustment is achieved by activating the body's natural self-healing capacities. Cranio-Sacral Therapy is beneficial both to reduce stress and improve general health. In addition, it also releases the full capacity of the brain's functioning while alleviating pain and pressure in the skull.

DEEP-TISSUE MUSCLE THERAPY

This scientific, systematic, individualized process induces elimination of toxic wastes, blockages and tension in fibrous connective tissue throughout the muscular structure. Effective Deep-Tissue Muscle Therapy provides therapeutic and curative effects not only for the affected areas and the rest of the anatomy but also for associated emotional and psychological conditions.

LYMPHATIC-DRAINAGE MASSAGE

A mode of therapy that stimulates the renewal of skin-tissue and regenerates the epidermis and its tissues. Lymphatic-Drainage Massage protects the body from infection and improves the functioning of its organs.

NEUROMUSCULAR MASSAGE

This deep-tissue therapy is designed to soothe the symptoms and alter the conditions of chronic pain. The masseuse uses hands, thumbs, forearms and elbows to provide brief, specific pressure to release muscle spasms and trigger points of radiating pain resulting in increased flexibility of both muscles and joints. Because it is an intense form of massage, this therapy is applied to a limited number of anatomical areas during any given session.

REFLEXOLOGY

One of the most popular, pleasant, healthful and effective forms of touch-therapy is reflexology— the art and science of foot and hand massage. It can be administered to oneself; but it is of much greater benefit when done by another. The pores at the soles of the feet are the largest in the body; so, they can absorb more quickly and more comprehensively both the oils and the electric impulses transmitted by reflexology. And, of course, the entire nervous system is connected to the clusters of nerves in the feet; therefore, proper foot massage sends immediate relief throughout the body.

ROLFING

This system of bodywork was originally called, "structural integration," and became 'Rolfing' because of Ida Rolf's, PhD more than 50 years of study, development and application. Dr. Rolf refined and simplified this process to three simple anatomical principles: 1. Almost every body is improperly aligned in some way, 2. Our best functioning happens when we are properly aligned with the Earth's gravitational field, and 3. The plasticity of our bodies allows for harmonious alignment at any age and under any condition. Rolfing involves ten sessions of education and rebalancing. For information about Rolfing — including a list of addresses and telephone numbers of certified Rolfers — go to **www.Rolf.org,** call **800-530-8875,** or write to **The Rolf Institute, 5055 Chaparral Court, Boulder, CO 80301**.

SCALP MASSAGE

The skillful application of Himalayan oils to the scalp relaxes and energizes the entire nervous system, nourishes brain-cells, and enriches the quality and texture of the hair. This procedure is part of the ancient, respected and proven Ayurvedic system of healing.

SHIATSU

This relaxing ancient Asian procedure is a form of acupuncture in which the fingers are used rather than needles to soothe the entire person, mind, body, emotions and spirit.

SKIN BRUSH MASSAGE

As its name indicates, this mode of massage involves the brushing of the skin to stimulate circulation, remove dead cells, and rejuvenate the skin. Results are that the skin is more taut and more vibrant in appearance, feeling and function.

SWEDISH THERAPEUTIC MASSAGE

Swedish Therapeutic Massage is a powerful means of reducing stress, fatigue and muscular discomfort. Long, soothing strokes produce full circulation of blood; kneading strokes stimulate the muscles and promote elimination of waste products; friction strokes stretch muscle attachments for improved range of motion.

THAI MASSAGE

Thai Massage is a unique form of acupressure that soothes the nervous system and facilitates its functioning. Deep, disciplined strokes similar to the movements in yoga stimulate the internal organs and realign the anatomy.

TRIGGER-POINT MASSAGE

Trigger-Point Therapy is also known as Neuromuscular Therapy and Myotherapy. The masseuse applies concentrated pressure to painful parts of the muscle that are called, "trigger-points," to calm spasms and aches.

BODY-AND-TOUCH-BASED THERAPIES

From the ancient practices of hydrotherapy, sweat lodges, saunas, Turkish baths, steam baths to name a few, cultures clearly understood the benefits of detoxifying the body. Modern medicine has borrowed from the wisdom of the ancients and, consequently, now utilizes hypothermia on cancer, microbes, and a broad array of both external and internal infections. Furthermore, far infrared applications are extensively utilized in the treatment of diseases that assault the immune system.

Beyond the therapeutic effects that these body-based medicinal procedures provide, each process relaxes and calms all of our systems as well as our mind, emotions and spirit. These additional benefits should contribute to your interest in these therapies.

ACU-POINTS (TSUBOTHERAPY)
Stimulates acupuncture points specifically related to body parts and organs.

ACUPRESSURE
Chinese system of massage more than 4,000-years-old. Uses the meridian points of acupuncture as touch therapy.

ACU-YOGA
Combines acupressure and yoga.

ALEXANDER TECHNIQUE
Teaches proper self treatment and self massage.

AMMA THERAPY
"Push-pull" therapy applying massage to painful areas by simply pushing and pulling them.

AMPAKU THERAPY
Diagnostic shiatsu massage for the abdominal region.

APPROPRIATE TOUCH (also called SAFE TOUCH or TRAUMA-TOUCH THERAPY)
Appropriate massage treatment to benefit those who have suffered sexual or other physical abuse.

AROMATHERAPY
The incorporation of essential oils in massage.

ARTHRO-KINETICS
Deepest and most powerful massage technique to treat joints and muscles.

AURA THERAPY
Non contact cleansing and stimulation of the body's electrical field by magnetic field application and other positive scientific influence.

BAREFOOT SHIATSU
Application of the fingers, palms and feet of the practitioner to the shiatsu points of the participant.

BINDEGEWEBSMASSAGE
Beneficial application for connective tissue.

BLADDER MERIDIAN
Asian bodywork applied to the 57 acupuncture points of this Yang meridian.

CHILDBEARING BODYWORK
Specific to the dynamic changes in a woman's body during pregnancy, labor and post-partum, benefiting both mother and child.

CAYCE/REILLY MASSAGE
Bodywork treatment created by the noted psychic, Edgar C. Cayce and Dr. Harold J. Reilly, the respected chiropractor and psychotherapist.

CHAIR MASSAGE
A very popular form of quick and accessible touch therapy where the participant sits in a massage chair.

CHI NEI TSANG (INTERNAL-ORGAN MASSAGE)
Internal organ massage to relieve obstructions of chi (the life-force).

CHUA KA
Self-administered bodywork system that can also include the guidance of a qualified practitioner.

CONNECTIVE TISSUE MASSAGE
Bodywork invigorating the circulatory and lymphatic systems.

CONSTITUTIONAL (HOLISTIC MASSAGE)
Assessment methodology and application to create a massage plan to suit each individual.

CORE BODYWORK
Multi-phase myofascial and structural somatic therapy.

CRANIAL SACRAL THERAPY
Gentle manipulation to locate and correct imbalances in the cranial-sacral region.

CRYSTAL/GEM HEALING
Gemstones placed on parts of the body in correspondence with primary energy fields.

CUPPING
Ancient technique using small jars to create a vacuum that alleviates diseased or injured parts of the body.

CYRIAX
Deep cross fiber friction massage.

DEEP TISSUE (DEEP MUSCLE)
Technique for the profound release of chronic pains and aches of muscles and connective tissues.

ESALEN
Slow, flowing strokes creating openness and a sense of ease (created at the Esalen Institute).

ETHERIC RELEASE
Body work system that relieves restricted emotional expression.

FACIAL (FACE-LIFT MASSAGE)
Rejuvenating the skin and muscles of the face without invasive and potentially scarring surgical techniques.

FASCIA (MYOFASCIA)
Touch treatment for tendons and the fibers that cover organs, nerves and blood vessels.

HAMA
Japanese massage technique based on shiatsu.

HAWAIIAN (LOMILOMI)
Traditional Hawaiian bodywork that has evolved to heal the participant and reconnect her with nature.

HELLERWORK
Eleven 90-minute sessions of deep-tissue bodywork, movement, education and dialogue designed to realign the body and release chronic tension and stress.

HOFFA TECHNIQUE
Five Swedish-massage strokes and pressure following the pattern of venous (toward the heart) blood flow.

ICE-THERAPY (CRYOTHERAPY)
The application of ice cold water therapeutically to localized areas of the body.

INFANT
Modified Swedish massage designed for babies aged 1-month to toddler.

JIN SHIN ACUTOUCH
Point touching on the body to stimulate the flow of chi throughout the meridians.

JIN SHIN DO: "The Way of the Compassionate Spirit" (BODY-MIND ACUPRESSURE)
Combines Japanese acupressure with the psychological theories of Wilhelm Reich and Carl Jung.

KINESIOLOGY
The science of mechanics and the principles of movement applied to touch therapy.

KRIPALU BODYWORK
Based on the principles of Kripalu Yoga, which emphasizes techniques that enhance awareness, deep relaxation, and meditative focus via touch therapy.

KRIYA
The intuition of the experienced practitioner appropriately applied to facilitate spontaneous energy flow during massage.

LYMPHATIC DRAINAGE (MANUAL LYMPH-DRAINAGE)
Connective tissue massage technique that accelerates the movement of lymphatic fluids, thereby reducing edema (accumulation of fluids) and congestion. It also cleanses the body and enhances immunity.

MCMILLAN TECHNIQUE
Medically applied Swedish massage strokes that facilitate the healing of maladies, diseases, infections and other conditions.

MEDICAL ORGONE THERAPY
Bodywork coupled with psychotherapy to liberate the self from its artificial psychological, emotional and physical self imposed constraints.

MENNELL TECHNIQUE
Massage using slow rhythms and light pressure on healthy tissue leading to touch-therapy treatment of damaged tissue.

NEUROMUSCULAR REPROGRAMMING (SOMA NEUROMUSCULAR INTEGRATION)
Ten-session system of body-mind therapy that provides both physical and psychological benefits. Gravity is used to promote the integration of the nervous system with other bodily systems, thereby increasing environmental awareness.

NAPRAPATHY
Traditional Czechoslovak touch therapy that relieves tension and promotes fluidity of motion.

NEURAL ORGANIZATION TECHNIQUE
Non-invasive application of massage to the anatomy to correct impairments and defects that create dysfunction in the nervous system.

OHASHIATSU
Traditional shiatsu (Japanese massage) system that incorporates psychological and spiritual dimensions of movement, exercise and meditation of Zen to generate ultimate harmonious balance of body/mind/emotion/spirit.

OKAZAKI RESTORATIVE (LONG-LIFE MASSAGE)
Based on the traditional seifukujitsu (restoration arts) system, combining touch healing with peaceful techniques of self-defense.

ORTHO-BIONOMY
Non-invasive osteo-therapeutically-based process to reduce stress, muscular fatigue and pressure on vital organs by positioning the participant's body in postures appropriate to the given condition.

THERESE PFRIMMER METHOD
Deep, penetrating system of corrective treatment, specifically designed to assist the restoration of damaged muscles and impaired soft tissue.

PILATES
A full body exercise system done either alone or with an experienced hands-on trainer. The process involves elongation of muscles and development of the abdomen, lower back and buttocks.

POLARITY-THERAPY
The electromagnetic energy patterns of the body are stimulated by bodywork. This system involves attention to diet, appropriate exercise, and psychological development.

POSTURAL INTEGRATION
Stimulating the connective tissue to release tension, thereby improving posture and aligning the skeletal structure properly, creating greater flexibility and facilitating free-flowing energy.

REBIRTHING
Gentle breathing technique to heighten self-awareness and stimulate the body's ability to heal itself. This process involves consultation, affirmations, and techniques and patterns of breathing that are often facilitated by the touch of a guide.

REFLEXOLOGY
(MASSAGE OF FEET AND HANDS) (ZONE-THERAPY)
Causes release of crystal deposits, thereby invigorating the nervous system and the meridian (electrical) system, thereby healing and balancing every organ of the body. *(Please see discussion and charts labeled, "Zone Therapy," in the chapter entitled, "Acupuncture without Needles".)*

REIKI
An ancient system of natural healing that uses biofields (the very energy of our bodies) to define the union of spiritual advancement and physical health. Ancient Tibetan monks from even more ancient Asian spiritual practices formalized it.

ROLFING (STRUCTURAL ALIGNMENT)
A unique ten-session system of bodywork that is designed to lengthen and redefine the matrix of the body's connective tissue to rejuvenate the participant physically, mentally, emotionally and even spiritually.

ROSEN METHOD
Promotion of self acceptance as a consequence of non-intrusive subtle touch, awareness of breathing, movement exercise, and harmonious sound.

RUSSIAN
The basic stroke forms of classical massage intensified to provide the least invasive and most comfortable treatment.

SACRO-OCCIPITAL TECHNIQUE (SOT)
An advanced gentle, yet corrective, chiropractic method emphasizing massage at the sacroiliac-joint.

SOMA NEUROMUSCULAR INTEGRATION (SOMA BODYWORK)
A ten-session system of body-mind therapy that generates systematic improvement of structural balance and integration of the nervous system, creating freedom of movement, spontaneity and creativity.

SOTAI
A unique method of generating muscular relaxation by inducing harmony of breath and movement.

SPINAL-TOUCH TREATMENT
A gentle-touch therapy that invigorates and balances the pelvis and spine, thereby improving posture, as well as eliminating pain and promoting health via muscular relaxation.

SWEDISH MASSAGE
This internationally respected system promotes circulation, relaxation and healing.

TANTSU (TANTRIC SHIATSU)
Watsu (water massage) techniques performed on land generating calmness, energy and awareness.

TEMPOROMANDIBULAR JOINT-THERAPY
Treatment of the jaw-joint via a variety of massage techniques to prevent and relieve TMJ.

THAI MASSAGE (NUAD BO-RARAN)
Ancient Asian system designed to release trapped energy and improve vitality by applying gentle pressure along the meridians.

THERAPEUTIC TOUCH
A contemporary mode derived from the ancient practice of direct energy healing through touch.

TIBETAN MASSAGE
The use of specific oils in massage to prevent illness and improve vitality and physical function.

TOUCH-FOR-HEALTH (APPLIED KINESIOLOGY)
Self applied pressurized touch to balance and strengthen weak muscles and promote the flow of energy to organs and glands.

TRIGGER-POINT THERAPY
The use of various methods to eliminate or heal trigger-points (areas of a given point of muscular pain).

UNTI
Bodywork and exercise used to maximize the skeletal system by combining soft-tissue evaluation and a specific method of light manual pressure to normalize muscles, tendons, ligaments and fascia, restoring balance to each individual musculature.

VIBRATIONAL HEALING MASSAGE-THERAPY
Profound, but gentle system to correct or eliminate physical, mental and emotional obstacles and imbalances.

VISCERAL MANIPULATION
Reinvigoration of the important physical, mental, emotional connections between the abdominal region and the entire body.

WATSU (WATER ZEN SHIATSU)
The application of bodywork upon an individual immersed in water, thereby creating a relaxing, releasing environment that liberates not only body but also mind, emotions and spirit.

WENGROW'S SYNERGY
Realignment of the natural vertical axis of the body.

ZERO-BALANCING
Comprehensive system unifying Western theories of anatomy with Asian theories of energy application.

NUTRIPUNCTURE

Nutripuncture, developed in France and utilized at **The Hippocrates Health Institute,** is another significant way to improve mind-body functioning. Nutripuncture is delivered orally; therefore, it mirrors acupuncture without resorting to needles, which are replaced by homeopathic medicine.

Throughout northern Europe, homeopathy has been an established form of healing for much more than a century. A poll conducted in France, for example, established that 40% of the population normally consumes homeopathic medicines. Similarly, 20% of all German allopathic practitioners prescribe homeopathic pills and tinctures routinely. The British population uses this natural mode of healing extensively and in Russia, with more than 500 physicians alone.

Interestingly, homeopathy is even more popular in India, with more than 100,000 homeopathic doctors nationwide. Increasing interest in natural healing has led to the greater use of homeopathics worldwide. Be sure to choose an experienced and sympathetic homeopathic physician who can suggest the best and safest medicine for your needs.

POSTURE

Our posture not only indicates but also affects our health, both physical and emotional. Stooped shoulders, a hunched back, and looking downward indicate lack of self-regard and low confidence. The secret to achieve proper posture is simple and threefold: first, live a healthy, fulfilled life that incorporates proper diet, exercise and rest; second, whenever you sit, do not slouch or bend; and third, when you stand or walk, elevate your chest and look forward. These natural means of maintaining posture will not only elevate your posture but also your mind and spirit.

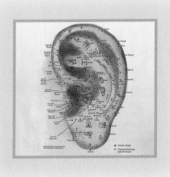

ELEVEN

Acupuncture Without Needles

Acupuncture and Acupressure are ancient systems of natural healing from Asia that access the body's bio-electric and bio-chemical pathways, called meridians. These systems restore balance and energy flow to the body. Traditional medicine believes that this energy force, called qi or chi, flows through the meridians and is the key to maintaining health and vitality. When chi energy is blocked, sickness and illness can result, but when chi is flowing, our bodies are harmonious and balanced and functioning well. These energy 'highways' are connected to specific organs and body functions through specific points. Acupuncture uses hair-thin needles and/or electrodes to stimulate the meridian points, while acupressure uses the same principles and meridian points, but works through finger pressure and massage rather than needles. By incorporating the following acupressure techniques, you can heal yourself naturally. At Hippocrates, we employ the best of Asian healing traditions with the best of non-invasive western technologies.

ACUPRESSURE

Acupressure is a complete and non-invasive ancient Chinese method of healing. It involves the strong yet soothing use of pressure against appropriate meridian points of the body to relieve pain. It is stimulating, yet calming. The meridians begin at the fingertips and tips of the toes and connect to the brain, which then delivers healing messages to the part of the body that needs it.

Acupressure increases and improves circulation, removes toxic wastes, relieves soreness, heals injuries, and minimizes labor pains. It also serves the whole person, body, mind, emotions, and spirit, by easing stress, fear and confusion and by reconnecting us with the essence or— "chi".

ZONE-THERAPY

Zone-therapy, also known as reflexology, has been a major part of traditional health and relaxation throughout the world. It involves the soothing therapeutic application of hands to zones or points on the hands and feet. Every part of the body is connected to at least one of these points. You can, of course, apply this therapy to yourself, hands to feet, and one hand to the other.

Apply finger pressure to those parts of hands and feet that affect the part of the body needing relief.

Stimulating every part of the body naturally, harmoniously and pleasantly not only feels good, but it also energizes that particular part of the body and the entire body as well. The words, "acupuncture," and, "acupressure," are more comforting when we realize that, "punct," means, "point"— the point at which the calming "pressure" is being applied.

Following are charts of acupressure points on the hand and throughout the body.

Hand Reflexology Chart

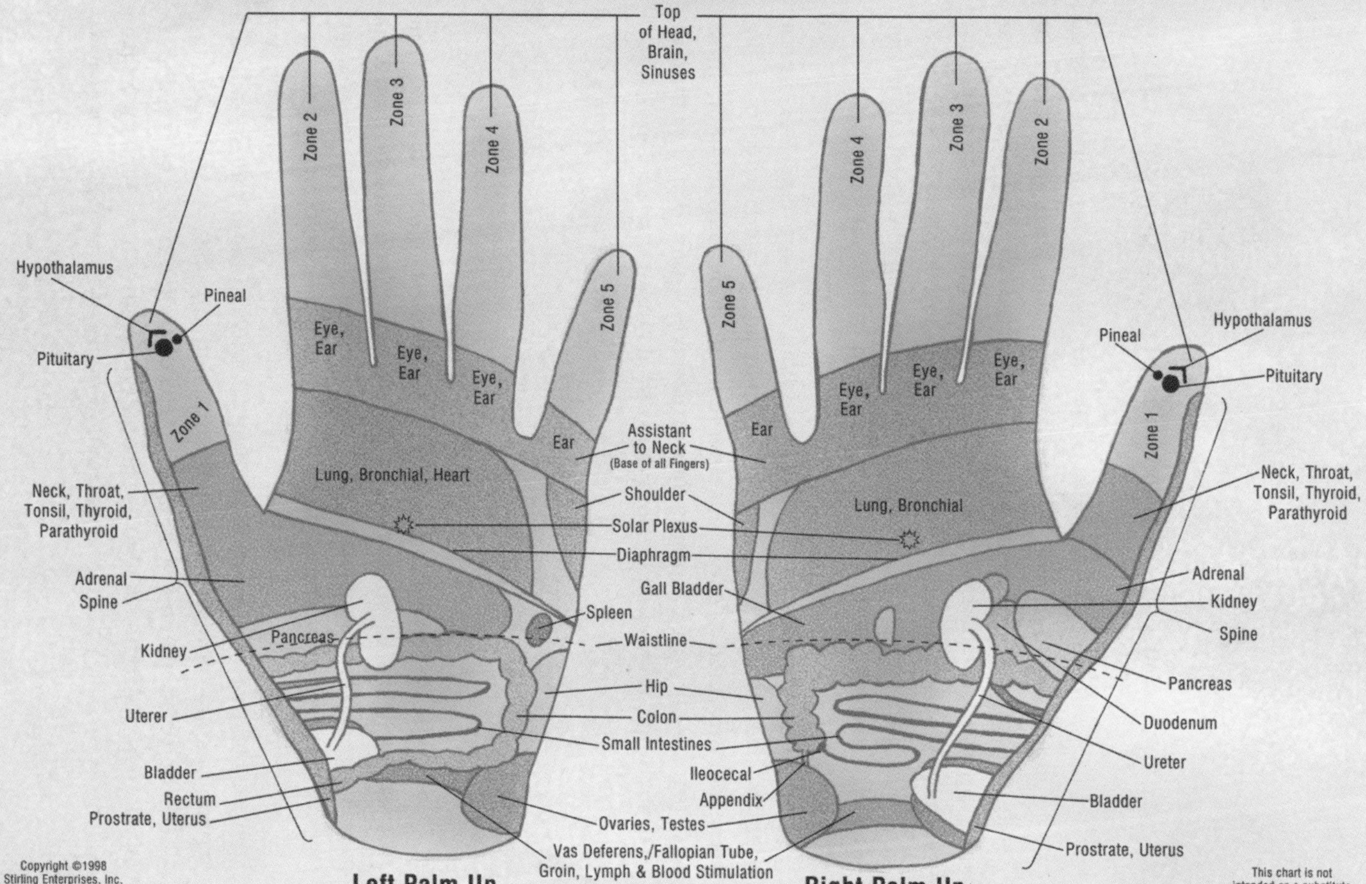

Left Palm Up

Right Palm Up

To help visualized reflexes on partners hands, turn chart upside-down.

This chart is not intended as a substitute for medical care.

Left Palm Up labels:
- Hypothalamus
- Pituitary
- Pineal
- Neck, Throat, Tonsil, Thyroid, Parathyroid
- Adrenal
- Spine
- Kidney
- Ureter
- Bladder
- Prostrate, Uterus
- Rectum
- Pancreas
- Zone 1
- Eye, Ear
- Eye, Ear
- Eye, Ear
- Ear
- Zone 2
- Zone 3
- Zone 4
- Zone 5
- Top of Head, Brain, Sinuses
- Lung, Bronchial, Heart
- Assistant to Neck (Base of all Fingers)
- Shoulder
- Solar Plexus
- Diaphragm
- Gall Bladder
- Waistline
- Spleen
- Hip
- Colon
- Small Intestines
- Ileocecal
- Appendix
- Ovaries, Testes
- Vas Deferens,/Fallopian Tube, Groin, Lymph & Blood Stimulation

Right Palm Up labels:
- Hypothalamus
- Pituitary
- Pineal
- Neck, Throat, Tonsil, Thyroid, Parathyroid
- Adrenal
- Kidney
- Spine
- Pancreas
- Duodenum
- Ureter
- Bladder
- Prostrate, Uterus
- Zone 1
- Zone 2
- Zone 3
- Zone 4
- Zone 5
- Eye, Ear
- Eye, Ear
- Eye, Ear
- Ear
- Lung, Bronchial

Foot Reflexology Chart

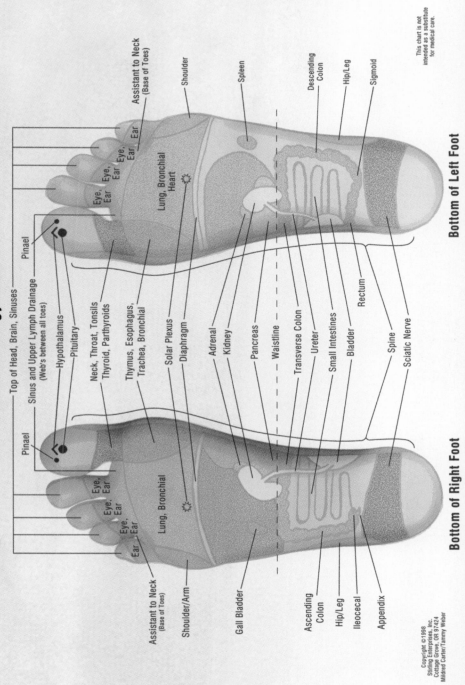

Top of Head, Brain, Sinuses

Sinus and Upper Lymph Drainage (Web's between all toes)

Pinael

Hypothalamus

Pituitary

Neck, Throat, Tonsils, Thyroid, Parthyroids

Thymus, Esophagus, Trachea, Bronchial

Solar Plexus

Diaphragm

Adrenal

Kidney

Pancreas

Waistline

Transverse Colon

Ureter

Small Intestines

Bladder

Rectum

Spine

Sciatic Nerve

Pinael

Eye, Ear

Eye, Ear

Eye, Ear

Ear, Ear

Assistant to Neck (Base of Toes)

Lung, Bronchial

Gall Bladder

Shoulder/Arm

Ascending Colon

Hip/Leg

Ileocecal

Appendix

Eye, Eye, Ear, Ear

Ear, Ear

Assistant to Neck (Base of Toes)

Shoulder

Lung, Bronchial Heart

Spleen

Descending Colon

Hip/Leg

Sigmoid

Bottom of Right Foot

Bottom of Left Foot

This chart is not intended as a substitute for medical care.

Ear-Organ Connection-Chart

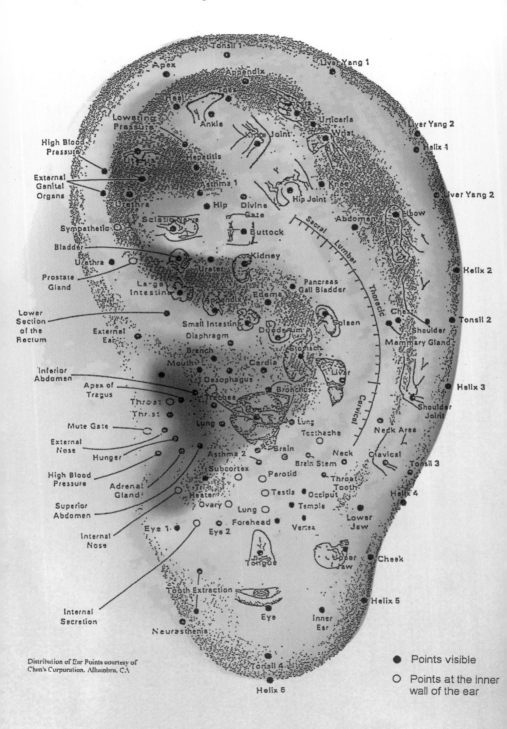

Distribution of Ear Points courtesy of
Chun's Corporation. Alhambra, CA

● Points visible

○ Points at the inner
wall of the ear

EAR-ACUPRESSURE

This mainstay of ancient Chinese medicine has been proven to combat and ease various illnesses and diseases as well as obesity, smoking, alcoholism, and other drug addictions.

The importance of the ears as part of the total body is stated in ***The Emperor's Classics of Internal Medicine***, published several thousands of years ago! The ear has more than 200 contact points, each of which embodies and conveys connections to every part of the body. Therefore, like the brain, heart, feet and hands, the ears are integrated parts of the whole. Proper treatment of the ears influences the health of the total person.

You can do this therapy easily for yourself. Hold the ear between your thumb and forefinger; use the forefinger to apply strong, but soothing pressure. Focus on a given area and apply strong but soothing pressure with your fingertips. When you feel uncomfortable, ease the contact and reapply gentler pressure. Ear acupressure is like pushing the buttons to start the flow of energy to and throughout various systems of your body. Take time every day to massage your ears for relief and rebalancing.

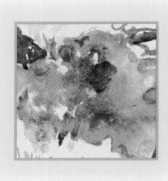

TWELVE

Magnetic Therapy

Magnetic therapies utilize the body's natural magnetic components (neurons, brain cells, red-blood cells, electrons, and the meridians— the electrical highway system of the body) without external electrical stimuli.

Magnets have been used for centuries throughout the world to address a variety of conditions and can be safely applied to every part of the body for 2-8 hours. Modern magnetic therapy involves the use of low-gauss manual magnets. They are similar to the magnets that you used as a child. They are placed on acupuncture points of the body to stimulate healing and reduce pain. When the electricity flows from one magnet to the other through your tissues, blockages and disorders are therapeutically addressed.

A double-blind study at Baylor University's Institute for Rehabilitation Research indicated that magnetic therapy alleviated pain in people recovering from polio. Magnetic therapy assists the body in dealing with headaches and other kinds of pain, growths, and blockages. Although you can use manual magnets at home, electromagnetic therapy and frequency-therapy are often applied clinically for thorough and faster remedy of more serious conditions.

ADVANCED ELECTROMAGNETIC THERAPY AND FREQUENCY-THERAPY

Electromagnetic therapy heals the body without invading it or harming it. Modern electromagnetic therapies combine technology with ancient healing that uses the meridian system. **Galvanic** and **Faradic** are among the most popular modern electromagnetic therapies. Another form of electrical therapy that relies on healing frequencies is **H-Wave**; it has been successfully used at The Institute for many years to overcome a variety of health concerns. The most frequently used form of electrical stimulation is **TENS—** **T**ranscutaneous **E**lectrical **N**erve-**S**timulation— in which a current is applied to the skin to control pain. The pattern of use usually follows acupuncture points.

Diathermia and **Magnetron** are just two types of electromagnetic therapies that have been used at The Institute to promote healing and results. The diapulse machine administers Diathermia. This powerful therapy was discovered during the early Twentieth Century. It is a non-thermal, high-frequency-pulsed, high-peak-powered electromagnetic energy. It has been researched and used to treat many conditions of disease and recovery. In Europe, this non-invasive technology is often prescribed for athletes to assist in recovery of damaged tissue after considerable exertion. It is also used extensively to regenerate nerve tissue (including spinal-cord injuries, trauma, burned tissue, and wounds), alleviate rheumatoid and osteo-arthritis, ulcers, edema in the brain, head wounds and coma, regulate renegade cells, and alleviate chronic headaches.

Magnetron uses complete circular electron interactivity to create intensified electromagnetic fields that stimulate cells to revert to their normal functioning. It has a low frequency, laser element that penetrates skin (tissue) non-invasively to re-energize sluggish cells and systems. Magnetron is used to purify and re-charge cells, reduce the pain of various conditions such as osteoporosis and arthritis, and heal wounds.

Vibrasan stimulates every system of the body by gently energizing the reclined body using vibration. This process separates unnaturally adhering cells from each other, relieving a condition called, "rouleau". When these cells are liberated from each other, they are able to return to normal functioning, absorbing more nutrients, creating stronger tissues and, most importantly, fighting damage caused by free radicals. This immune-boosting therapy helps to prevent and eliminate many disorders.

Hydrosonic — also known as "Cross Brain-wave Treatment" — is based on a therapeutic combination of harmonious sound, water and vibrational frequencies. A waterbed is placed above a large, sophisticated, bed-like system of speakers so that the participant's body can relax while the auditory senses are applied. This process releases brain hormones and endorphins that stimulate the brain stem, which connects the nervous system to the brain. This therapeutic stimulus assists in the development of immune system cells; it is used successfully for insomnia, dyslexia, ADD, nervousness, hyperactivity, stress, and anxiety.

As always, please consult a qualified local practitioner about the use of these and other electromagnetic therapies.

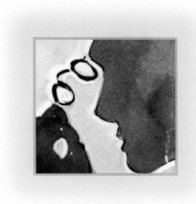

THIRTEEN

Things Look Better If You See Better: Improving Your Vision

The importance of sight is obvious. The eyes are used to convey many things about life: awareness, for example, when we say, "I see," rather than "I understand;" proof when we say, "seeing is believing;" and to the presence of truth when we say, "open your eyes!" And, how often do we say, "the eyes are the mirror of the soul." But, sadly, our eyes and vision suffer from many problems, from genetic issues, to environmental hazards, to accidents. Furthermore, one of the worst aspects of aging is the loss of vision. Fortunately, natural home healing can fight these problems.

Our eyes consist primarily of two very basic elements: they are 65% water and 35% protein; the eyes have more protein than any other body part. They also have the highest percentage of potassium, as well as high amounts of Vitamin C and glutathione. These essential components of our eyes can be nurtured and protected in a very basic way. First, we must eat healthfully, especially foods that are rich in beta-carotene; and, we must protect our eyes from both internal and external hazards.

"Food for thought," is good for the mind; food for sight is good for both the mind and the body. It is real and physically nourishing, like the Aloe Vera; Ginkgo Biloba and Zinc. Furthermore, topical applications of eye-bright, Vitamin C, riboflavin, bilberry-water, and strained wheatgrass-juice have been effective in healing the eyes and improving vision.

There are many physical, chemical, mechanical and electrical visual hazards in our environment. So, we must wear glasses or goggles to protect us. Use protective eyewear to shield your eyes from UV rays when the sun is too strong, when you work or play outside, or enjoy hobbies or sports of any sort that might jeopardize your eyes. Those who live in the sun belt develop twice as many cataracts as people who live in less sun-drenched climates. Modern life demands much more of our eyes than ever. Consider the fact that we (and especially children) view television and computer monitors for many hours per day.

Your eyes, like other parts of your body, benefit from exercise. I have used and recommended **The W. D. Bates Eye-Method** both at Brandal and Hippocrates. Doctor Bates was a progressive healer who used and prescribed proper nutrition, exercise and relaxation as the cornerstones of health. This gifted ophthalmologist created a system of exercise for the eyes. It consists primarily of all natural healthy movements for the eyes in coordinated sequences. Proper eye exercise has been proven to improve and sustain vision to such a great extent as to eliminate the need for glasses and to limit the decline of vision that generally accompanies aging and diseases such as diabetes.

As important as it is to keep our eyes open to see and to understand, it is equally important to close them in order to rest and to restore them. This means that we must close our eyes safely and restfully as often as possible, not only during sleep but also for meditation, prayer, naps, and other restful pauses during our busy days. Eyes are also very prone to fatigue, making sufficient sleep a top priority. Eyes that are fatigued are sore and less able to function, which compromises our work and play, and, more seriously, our safety. When we are driving or engaged in other potentially dangerous activity it is essential that we have clear vision and are of a clear mind.

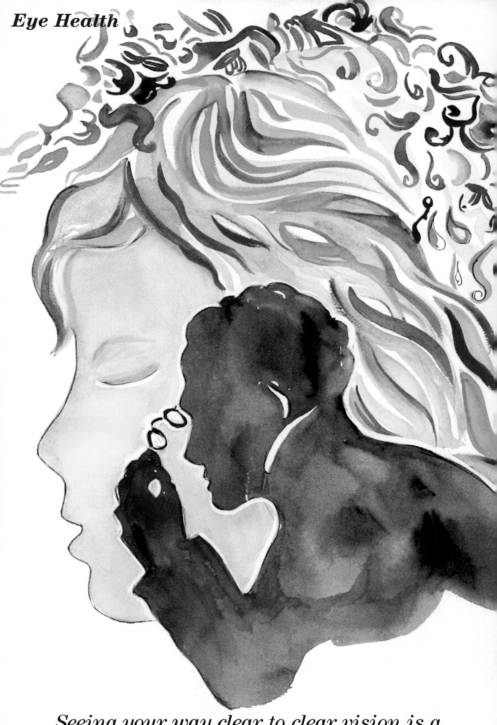

Seeing your way clear to clear vision is a rewarding and healthy endeavor.

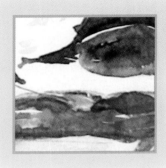

FOURTEEN

Conclusion

We have all heard the expression, "hearth and home". Now, having made our journey through this book, we can add this important phrase, "health at home". As you have learned, you can successfully and easily care for yourself and your family's health at home. And, what better and more logical place to do it?

Just as the house is the home of the body, the body is the home of the mind, the emotions and the spirit. So, while we are securing the health of our bodies within our homes, we are also ensuring our mental, emotional and spiritual health.

That is the inner reality. We also have an equally greater need to attend to our larger homes— our community, our environment, our world, and our universe— our shared home. And, we do that by living our best in our bodies in our homes.

Responsibility is rewarding. As we care for ourselves, our immediate and extended family, and our environment, we make the world a better

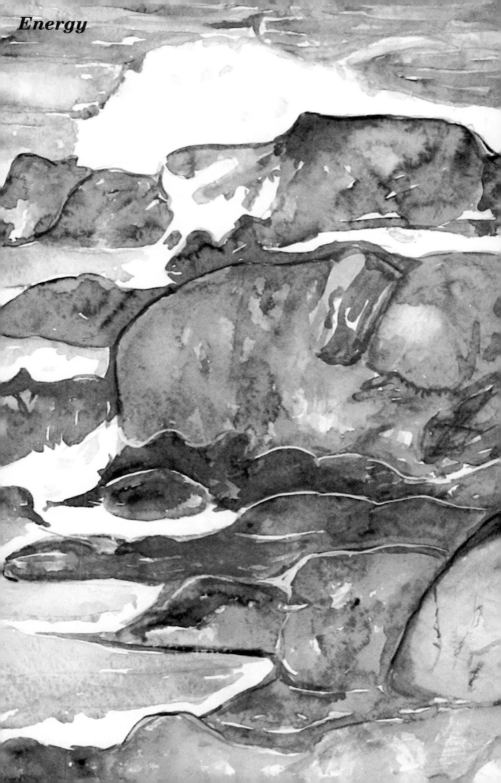

Energy

place. Reliance on questionable institutions and false "experts" undermines our natural order and creates chaos in our homes and our lives. Let us aspire to be our best, so that everything that we do contributes rather than detracts. Simple acts of help and healing not only mend our wounds but also shape our lives and the lives of others.

Those of us who have the honor of influencing others must have the strength to direct our own lives positively as well. We are all in the process of healing, and we all face new challenges daily; these challenges can be constructive when we use them to grow.

Nature provides us with everything that we need to live a happy and healthy life. Welcome nature back into our homes and our lives: walk and look at the scenery rather than sitting and watching television; listen to the sound of nature, rather than talk on the phone; and use your legs rather than the car.

When we say "hearth and home," we mean essentially that the heart is in the home. And, when our hearts are in our homes, we have the best opportunity for health. So, put your heart into your life and your home, and both will be filled with loving health.

(For more-detailed discussion of various subjects considered in this book, please see *__LifeForce__* by Brian Clement and George Kovacs, *__Living Food for Optimum Health__*, and the other fine books in **The Hippocrates Series**.)

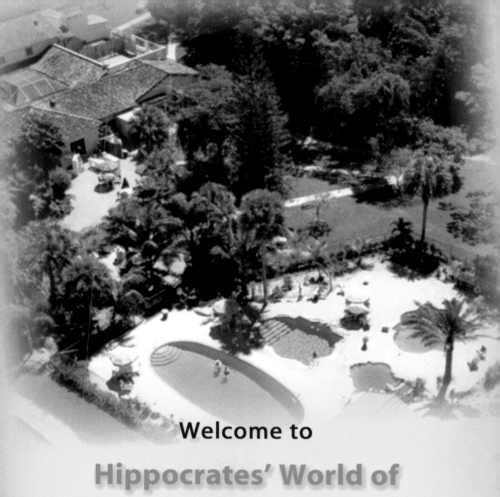

Welcome to

Hippocrates' World of Life Change Programs, products and services…

the place to renew your body, your spirit and your mind

www.HippocratesInstitute.org

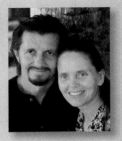

Welcome and thank you for taking time to explore how the Hippocrates Programs, products and services can enrich your life and the lives of others. For 50 years, we have served hundreds of thousands of people in their journey back to health. Our philosophy is based on the belief that a pure enzyme-rich diet, proper exercise, positive thinking and non-invasive therapies are the essential elements of optimum health and vibrant living. Join us and our wonderful staff and faculty and learn for yourself why *Spa Magazine* ranked Hippocrates Health Institute the #1 Medical Wellness Spa in the World and how you can reclaim your birthright of extraordinary health and well-being.

Brian and Anna Maria Clement

Our commitment is to provide the finest natural health technologies from around the globe in a meditative and healing setting. In addition to delicious organic living foods, everyone who stays at Hippocrates receives their very own personally-designed program incorporating some of the most highly specialized and effective therapies available today: ozonated pools, infrared saunas, electro-magnet & Vibrosaun treatments, Diapulse & Hyperbaric Oxygen therapies, Wheatgrass & Juice therapies, Dark Field Analysis, and personal consultations with nutrionists, medical doctors and other health experts, as well as meditation & yoga. The experience will astound you!

*"Longevity in and of itself is not the goal, rather it is **living well throughout your life** that matters most."* –Brian Clement

Our desire to enjoy a long, healthy and fulfilling life is brought to fruition by nurturing ourselves on each level, mentally, emotionally, spiritually and physically and throughout every experience of life. Life is a process of learning, the essence of which requires an open mind and the ability to choose; when you see learning as an expansion of yourself that provides vast and potentially endless new opportunities for happiness and success, both learning and life become easier and more rewarding.

To achieve an enlightened and enriched grand age, one must also have a purpose to live, an ultimate and definitive goal that is the foundation for our daily pursuits. Nutrients, movement, positive attitude, pure thoughts and spiritual openness are just some of the tools required to achieve great longevity; yet, no one of these tools individually has the strength to propel you to a desired status. Together, though, they are the mechanics of longevity. To extend our lives, we must have a passionate desire for fulfillment, tapping into our vital energies daily to create ease, grace, health, and happiness...for many, many years.

HIPPOCRATES LIFE CHANGE PROGRAMS

3-WEEK LIFE CHANGE PROGRAM

Our signature program provides our guests with the necessary tools to take control of their own personal well-being and to allow the body to maximize its potential and heal itself in a natural way. As our guest, you receive a comprehensive introduction to the Hippocrates Lifestyle and the bio-science behind the miracle stories of Hippocrates. The Life-Change Program not only features the specifics of the diet, but also includes experiences of many therapies such as massage, colon hydrotherapy and the psychology of wellness. You also learn tips for beginning and maintaining this lifestyle at home. **The Hippocrates Life Change Program begins every Sunday and ends on a Saturday, and is offered continuously throughout the year. One week is the minimum stay and three weeks is the entire program.**

THE HEALTH EDUCATOR PROGRAM
9-Week Life Change Program

Do you want an extensive education in the Living Foods Lifestyle? Do you wish to teach others about the Hippocrates program? Do you desire to add the knowledge of living foods nutrition and other integrated disciplines to your current career? If yes, the Hippocrates Health Educator Program is the comprehensive educational experience in the Living Foods Lifestyle that you desire. **This 9-week Professional Program is offered three times per year in the Spring, Summer and Fall.**

SAVE YOUR LIFE! LECTURE SERIES

Last Thursday of every month at Hippocrates Health Institute.

- An invaluable introduction to the Hippocrates' Living Foods Lifestyle: Learn how to increase energy, and build strength and vitality
- Hear valuable strategies for creating better health and for preventing and recovering from threatening illnesses from world
- Enjoy a complimentary Hippocrates' buffet dinner!

For information and reservations on any of these programs call 800.842.2125 or visit our website www.HippocratesInstitute.org

The Hippocrates Health Series...

Bring the Life Change Experience Into Your Home!

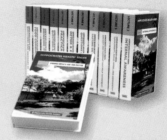

This extraordinary tape series will introduce you to the foundation of successful living and the principles of the Hippocrates Program, that have consistently proven to restore vitality and improve the quality of life. The secrets of creating optimal health are now yours to enjoy at home! Just some of the topics covered in this comprehensive series are:

- Digestion and elimination
- Supplements, Algae, Herbs and Homeopathy
- Food Combining
- Fasting
- Emotional and spiritual healing
- Detoxification

Plus! Your questions about the science and psychology of this program and why it works, and much, much more…

Available on DVD, VHS, CD and Audio Cassette or by calling 800.842.2125

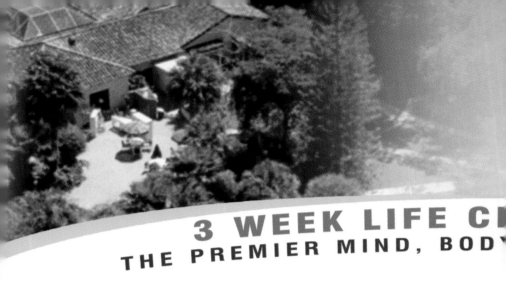

3 WEEK LIFE CH
THE PREMIER MIND, BODY

For 50 years our *Life Change Program* has provided tens of thousands of people from around the world the knowledge they need to optimize health. Our guests are fortifying their health, recovering from life-threatening illnesses, finding more peace, joy and balance in their lives and experiencing more happiness and vibrancy than ever before. Now you can too!

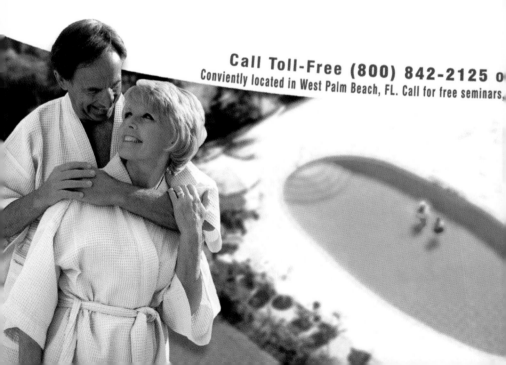

Call Toll-Free (800) 842-2125 o
Conviently located in West Palm Beach, FL. Call for free seminars,

Products for a Healthier Life...

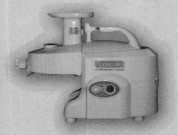
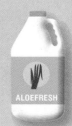
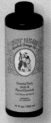
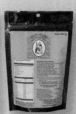

Hippocrates Living Food Processor

Finally, an easy to use juicer/living foods processor that is functional with every aspect of the Hippocrates Living Foods Program. The Hippocrates Living Food Processor handles all of your juicing needs, as well as creating everything from nut pates to banana ice cream and it comes with a 12-year warranty!

LifeGive Aloe

This unique aloe, grown in coral rock, is used for a wide variety of purposes. Everything from digestion to chronic health challenges have benefited from this powerful sun soaked plant extract.

Brain/Body Powder and Brain/Body Oil

A new and exciting body of evidence has surfaced on the positive effects of fatty acids and specific berries on brain function. Now, you can benefit from this exclusive and proprietary formula, comprised of hemp, flax, cranberry and black raspberry, that not only provides the best form of Omega 3, 6s & 9s, but all of the essential amino acids, which are critical for building muscle fiber!

Introducing...

The Hippocrates Series of *LifeGive* Products!

LIFEGIVE: WOMEN'S FORMULA

A "woman's" general rejuvenation and female organ supporting formula to support "femininity", beauty, endocrine and hormonal balance. Condition specific for PMS, and other imbalances. Strengthening of the female physiology. This is a "must" daily formula for every pre-menopausal woman.

HHI-ZYME - Digestive Aid

Attain optimum health with our own improved, time tested formula. Provides essential nutrients, vitamins, minerals and enzymes to enhance digestion of foods. This highly active, potent blend minimizes metabolic stress.

LIFEGIVE PAR-A-GONE

A traditional herbal formula for the elimination of parasites (worms, amoebas, others) and for associated parasitic conditions including dysentery. May be taken in advance of travel for prevention of acquiring parasites. Also useful during travel.

LIFEGIVE REVITALIFE - Recovery Formula

Feel alive again! Specially designed for rejuvenation and restoration of strength and energy. All natural herbal concentrate contains enzymes and oxygen.

These are just a few samples of hundreds of health-giving products available at Hippocrates' Store. All of these products are available by calling Hippocrates' Store at 561.471.8876 Ext. 102 or 103. Store Hours: Monday to Friday 9am – 5pm & Saturday 9am – 3pm American E.S.T.

You know why we're smiling?

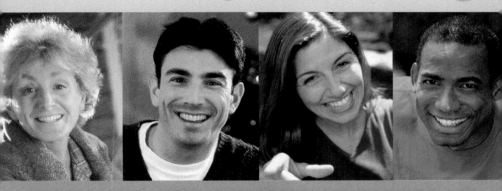

...because we love what we do! The 9-week Health Educator Program at Hippocrates Health Institute gave us the confidence, the experience and the education that we needed to establish a successful career as a health educator."

HEALTH EDUCATION

Enzymatic Nutrition
Anatomy & Physiology
Yoga & Basic Massage
Physical Fitness
Live-Food Preparation
Life Coaching Skills
Live-Cell Microscopy
Sprouting & Composting
Natural Therapies
Basic Counseling
The Science of Living Foods
Public Speaking
Reflexology
Iridology

BUSINESS EDUCATION

Marketing & PR Essentials
Partnership vs. Proprietorship
Creating a successful business plan
Tax and accounting basics
Incorporating your business
Working with barter exchanges
Negotiating with vendors
Acquiring startup capital

Call today and enroll (561) 471-8876
www.hippocratesinst.com

Health Educator Program at Hippocrates Health Institute

Other books and publications from Hippocrates Health Institute

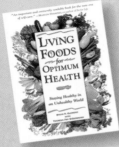

Living Foods for Optimum Health
By Brian Clement, Ph.D., N.M.D.

An introduction to the lifestyle that has helped hundreds of thousands of people overcome chronic diseases such as cancer, diabetes, heart disease, chronic fatigue syndrome & fibromyalgia, arthritis, candidiasis, depression, and more to lead fulfilling and happy lives. The first book from one of the world's foremost authorities on the Living Foods Lifestyle.

Healthful Cuisine
By Anna Maria Clement, Ph.D., N.M.D. and Kelly Serbonich, Living Foods Chef

A volume of raw, living food vegetarian recipes from the world's leading medical wellness spa, *Hippocrates Health Institute*. This easy-to-use food preparation guide will satisfy even the most discriminating of chefs. Spiral binding and coated pages make it a favorite in any kitchen!

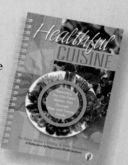

LifeForce *Coming Soon!*
By Brian Clement, Ph.D., N.M.D.

Understand how living thoughts and living foods create subtle energy flow that is the source of all creation and longevity. Learn what 50 years of research from the world's #1 Medical Wellness Spa proves: we can generate lifeforce to achieve infinitely higher levels of health and well-being.

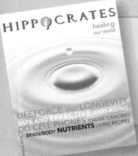

Subscribe FREE Today!

Join the thousands who have achieved greater health through the Hippocrates Life Change Programs. Call toll free 1.800.842.2125 or 561.471.8876 to order your *FREE subscription* to Hippocrates Health Institute's Quarterly Magazine.

HIPP**⚕**CRATES
HEALTH INSTITUTE

1443 Palmdale Court • West Palm Beach, FL 33411
www.HippocratesInstitute.org

Hippocrates is a 501(c)(3) non-profit educational organization and a 70-room in-resident facility located in West Palm Beach, FL with a lifelong mission to educate people on how to live a vibrant and healthy life. This *Marketing Awareness Profile* is a patent pending product of Healthfulcommunications.com

NOTES